man
to
man

man to man

John Chesterman and Michael Marten

PADDINGTON PRESS LTD

NEW YORK & LONDON

Library of Congress Cataloging in Publication Data
Chesterman, John.
  Man to Man.
  1. Men – Health and hygiene. 2. Men – Sexual
behavior. I. Marten, Michael, joint author.
II. Title.
RA777.8.C48   613'.04'23   78–8292
ISBN 0 7092 0512 0
ISBN 0 448 22681 2 (U.S. and Canada only)

Filmset in England by Servis Filmsetting Ltd., Manchester
Printed and bound in the United States
Designed by Sandra Shafee
IN THE UNITED STATES
PADDINGTON PRESS
Distributed by
GROSSET & DUNLAP

IN THE UNITED KINGDOM
PADDINGTON PRESS

IN CANADA
Distributed by
RANDOM HOUSE OF CANADA LTD.

IN SOUTHERN AFRICA
Distributed by
ERNEST STANTON (PUBLISHERS) (PTY.) LTD

IN AUSTRALIA AND NEW ZEALAND
Distributed by
A.H. & A.W. REED

Contents

Appearance

We live "inside" our bodies and personalities. They are ours to use, and we would be foolish not to be aware of them. But awareness is one thing, and anxiety is another. The one sure way to stack the odds against you is to worry about yourself. Worry will make you ugly, ill and unsuccessful.

Don't worry about your faults. Either do something about them, turn them to advantage, or forget them.

There is no such thing as a "normal" or "average" person. We are all different, thank goodness.

Everyone is sexually attractive to someone. There are even some women who go for over-groomed, musclemen stereotypes.

When in doubt, change your habits, loosen up, get out of your rut, experiment, take a few chances and do something different, if only in one small area of your life. Boredom is your fault.

Don't let anyone set your targets for you. Do it yourself. Have no faith in advertising, aerosols or instant cures . . . unless you do it for fun.

And, if possible, always do it for fun.

WEIGHT AND HEIGHT

I'm worried about my height. Is there any way to increase it?

"You're not so very tall," Lauren Bacall tells Humphrey Bogart in *The Big Sleep.*

"Next time," Bogey replies, "I'll come in a morning suit, wear a pair of stilts and carry a tennis racket."

Apart from the medieval rack, there is no known way of increasing your physical height. On the other hand, there are severals ways of *appearing* taller. The most important is posture. A man can lose as much as 2–3 inches by slouching. Bad posture is a bad habit that is difficult to break. Regular exercises help. Stand straight, with your shoulders squared, and your stomach held in. Sit straight too. Secondly, wear clothes that are tight-fitting to accentuate height and slenderness. Thirdly, stay slim; portliness makes you look smaller. Finally, wear high heels or platform shoes.

When all this is said and done, you may still be below average height. But there is nothing further you can do about it. Worrying only compounds the problem. Tallness is *not* a prerequisite for social success.

Is it true that one gets smaller as one grows older?

Yes. Your spine becomes slightly shorter in old age because of deterioration of the vertebral disks. More important, weakening of your body muscles means that you can't hold yourself as erect as before. The combined loss of physical height and good posture will make you at least 2–3 inches shorter.

Does the 95-lb. weakling really miss out?

If you go around thinking of yourself as a 95-lb. weakling, the chances are that you will indeed miss out – not because of your weight, height and strength (or lack of them), but because you have adopted an image of yourself that is bound to sap your confidence. It's as if one of the Charles Atlas figures at the other end of the muscle spectrum went around thinking of himself as a 250-lb. monster, blushing and cringing whenever a girl looked at him.

The first thing to get straight is that your physical appearance is *not* the only, and not even the most important, determinant of how attractive you are to the opposite sex. Kindness, generosity, humor, intelligence, energy – all can count for as much as physique; often, they are far more important.

The second point is that opinion polls have found that most women nowadays are *not* attracted to the extravagantly muscled figure of the traditional he-man. What they find most attractive is a small, tight ass.

How much should I weigh?

The table below indicates *roughly* how much you should weigh if you are twenty-five or older and of more or less medium build. The problem with insurance company statistics is that they are averages, and averages tend to disguise nature's variety. Some people have a naturally heavier build. Others, such as professional wrestlers and weightlifters, may be heavier because of the muscles they have built up. However, if you are more than 15–20 lbs. heavier than the figure given below for your height, you are probably overweight whatever your build.

HEIGHT IN BARE FEET	DESIRABLE WEIGHT (in indoor clothing)
5ft 1in	118–129 lbs
5ft 2in	121–133
5ft 3in	124–136

5ft 4in	127–139
5ft 5in	130–143
5ft 6in	134–147
5ft 7in	138–152
5ft 8in	142–156
5ft 9in	146–160
5ft 10in	150–165
5ft 11in	154–170
6ft	158–175
6ft 1in	162–180
6ft 2in	167–185
6ft 3in	172–190

(Source: Metropolitan Life Insurance Company)

Should I be worried about being overweight?

Extra weight places an added burden on all the functions of your body and, as insurance company statistics confirm, shortens your lifespan. Hippocrates knew this two thousand years ago. "Persons who are naturally very fat," he wrote, "are apt to die earlier than those who are slender." According to one modern estimate, a man who weighs 185 lbs when he should weigh 140 lbs has his life expectancy shortened by four years. Specific problems are:

Excessive fat in your body adds to your chances of getting diabetes, gall stones, kidney disease, high blood pressure, pneumonia and cirrhosis of the liver.

Excessive weight adds to your chances of getting arthritis (from strain on the joints), hernias, varicose veins, and broken bones. It also contributes to problems following surgery.

The answer to the question is that you shouldn't worry about being overweight, you should do something about it. Some people, of course, may prefer to eat well and die younger. For others, the effort in staying slim may just possibly take as great a physical and psychic toll as remaining fat.

Are some people naturally inclined to getting fat?

If two people eat and exercise the same amount, one may grow round and heavy while the other stays lean and slender. The difference seems to lie in the metabolism. Food provides your body with fuel (in the form of proteins, fat and carbohydrates) which is burned up in the course of your daily activity. It's when you consume more fuel than you burn that problems arise. What happens to the surplus? If you're an "ectomorph," your metabolism speeds up automatically so that the surplus gets burned however inactive you are. Ectomorphs tend to remain skinny however much they eat. "Endomorphs," on the other hand, have a less flexible metabolism; their surplus fuel is stored in the body as fat. To avoid getting fat, the endomorph has no choice but to eat less or exercise more, and preferably both.

What makes you an ectomorph or endomorph is uncertain, but the tendency appears to be inherited.

How can I lose weight?

Every year a hundred effortless and brand-new techniques for getting slim are touted around. The fact remains that there are just two ways of losing weight: eating less and doing more.

Eating less All genuine weight-reducing diets restrict the number of calories you consume, whether by reducing your overall consumption of food or by changing your diet from high- to low-calorie foods. A variety of weight-reducing diets are to be found in books on dieting including low-calorie cookbooks. If you're uncertain which diet to adopt, or have tried in the past and failed, consult a doctor.

There are a number of aids to dieting including substitute or alternative foods, and drugs. Substitute foods include low-calorie bread, "diet" colas, skim milk, and saccharin as a replacement for sugar. (The US Food and Drugs Administration (FDA) is currently trying to ban saccharin as a suspected cause of cancer.) Drugs in the form of slimming or diet pills are usually amphetamine-based. They work by reducing your appetite, but can lead to addiction if taken regularly.

Obesity is rampant in the rich industrialized nations because people are eating more and exercising less. A recent US government survey showed that both men and women had, on average, gained 14 lbs in weight compared to what was average in the 1960s. The executive who eats a healthy breakfast, sits in his office all morning, enjoys a large lunch, then sits in his office all afternoon, and ends up with a few cocktails and a substantial dinner, is simply not doing enough to justify the amount he eats. Worry and responsibility do *not* burn up food-fuel. One answer is to cut out a meal entirely and replace it with some other form of relaxation.

Doing more People who lead active physical lives rarely become fat. But people who lead sedentary lives rarely lose weight by exercise alone. One problem is that exercise not only burns up the calories but also increases your appetite. Eating more after vigorous exercise won't make you slimmer. One author notes that a single business lunch can nullify the effects of a nonstop, eight-hour game of squash. The fact is that you have to take an enormous amount of exercise in order to lose weight – a seven-hour swim or a fifty-mile walk will burn off only one pound.

Exercise, therefore, is almost useless unless performed in combination with a slimming diet. With a diet, however, it is extremely valuable, contributing to your health and fitness as well as to any weight loss. It's also important to realize that regular small amounts of exercise, such as a half-hour walk or ten-minute jog every day, are more valuable than occasional bouts of extremely strenuous activity, such as a weekly game of squash or long-distance run.

How can I avoid fraudulent methods of dieting?

Any method of dieting that doesn't reduce the number of calories you consume or increase your activity is almost certainly a fraud. There are more myths about losing weight than can be individually described here, but several of the most common are as follows:

Though much of your body consists of water, drinking less fluids or sweating more will not reduce your weight in the long term. If you go thirsty for days, you'll certainly lose weight, but you will also remain dehydrated until you replace the lost fluid. Water isn't fat. It's the same story if you swelter in a Turkish bath or exercise in a rubber suit. What *is* effective is to stop drinking high-calorie liquids like whisky, gin and vodka, or high-carbohydrate ones like beer and cider, and replace them with soft drinks or water.

Other myths include suggestions that you will lose weight by eating less salt, drinking no coffee, and changing from sugar to honey or glucose.

It is also untrue that you will lose weight by eating heavy meals so that you'll stop nibbling in between, or by nibbling in between so that you'll eat less at meals.

Massage is also a useless slimming technique. It may make you glow with feelings of health and fitness, but it would require so great a pressure to break up your fat cells that your tissues would be irretrievably damaged. Similarly, "passive" exercise machines that "exercise" you with vibrating belts will rub you and cost you but won't dissolve any fat. They won't even tone up your muscles much.

Finally, special garments which mold your figure and are often claimed to "melt your fat away" will do the former but not the latter. Forcible redistribution of fat is not the same as loss of weight. It also tends to be uncomfortable.

13

FITNESS

What is fitness?

Fitness can be defined as a person's ability to function at a high level of physical efficiency. Whereas machines wear out the more they are used, organic systems like the human body grow in strength, endurance and flexibility with increased exercise. Getting fit is a matter of extending your physical capabilities. Below a certain level of daily activity, these capabilities degenerate through disuse: muscles become flabby; heart and lungs are unable to cope with sudden or prolonged exertion; and balance, coordination and reaction time all suffer.

Modern industrial society encourages an essentially sedentary lifestyle. Hard physical activity has for many become an optional rather than an integral part of life. Like the person who has been bedridden so long he can barely stand, urban man is often a physical weakling whose adaptability and endurance are strictly limited.

Physical fitness consists of three interrelated elements: strength, endurance and general work capacity. Strength is the ability to exert muscular force. Endurance is the ability to exert force (or withstand strain) over a period of time. General work capacity is the overall efficiency of the body, and particularly its ability to supply itself with enough energy and oxygen to maintain required levels of activity. Since this depends on the efficiency of the heart-lung system, it is often referred to as "circulo-respiratory" or CR fitness.

Physical fitness is, of course, relative. There is no absolute level of fitness, and the level you need to achieve will depend largely on your environment and lifestyle. A mountaineer or champion athlete needs to maintain a level of fitness that is quite unnecessary for the average office worker.

What are the benefits of fitness?

Physical fitness is not a panacea which will cure all your ills, but it certainly contributes to your health and, other things being equal, adds to your energy and lifespan.

A fit body is in every sense a stronger body. It resists infection more effectively, and recovers more rapidly when you do fall ill. It is able to exert itself for longer periods with less strain. And it performs more efficiently – burning up fewer calories in a given activity than an unfit body.

Muscles, including the heart, are strengthened by regular exercise. They become larger, more powerful and more flexible. An athlete's heart is on average almost 20 percent larger than a sedentary worker's. It pumps more blood per stroke, and is therefore able to operate at a lower heart rate – 55–65 beats per minute compared to a sedentary person's 75–85. Increased blood flow also improves the efficiency of your cardio-vascular system and reduces your chances of suffering from heart disease.

Another benefit of stronger muscles is improved posture. This not only improves your appearance, but also your appetite and digestion. And it reduces the chances of backache.

Fitness tends to increase physical and mental alertness. Your reactions are faster, your movements better coordinated and more finely judged. You are likely to fell an increased sense of well-being, with deeper sleep and more energy when awake. This isn't just a psychological reaction. Because your body functions more efficiently when you're fit, you get more energy out of a given quantity of food-fuel than someone who is less fit, and you use that energy more effectively.

Does physical fitness contribute to psychological well-being?

It is only in western countries that a sharp division is seen between body and mind. Oriental exercise systems such as yoga and the martial arts are simultaneously physical and psychological (or spiritual), and are designed to act upon the body-mind as an integrated whole. From this point of view, a man who develops his body while ignoring his mind (or vice versa) is as unbalanced as a man who develops the muscles of one leg while ignoring those of the other.

Being physically fit will tend to enhance your mental alertness and may give you an overall sense of well-being. But it will not, by itself, cure any psychological problems you may have. From the eastern viewpoint, being physically fit is only one part of being a fit person.

How much exercise do I need to get and stay fit?

Becoming fit requires more effort than maintaining a given level of fitness. Just how much effort will depend on such factors as how unfit you are to start with, how rapidly you want to get fit, and your age, weight and general health. Depending on your consumption, cigarettes and alcohol can double the effort required.

Basic get-fit routines recommended by different instructors and books vary widely, but the following is standard:

Walking Start by walking one mile a day in fifteen minutes (4 mph). Gradually, without straining or exhausting yourself, build up to three miles a day in thirty-nine minutes.

Stationary running Start with one minute a day at a rate of 70–80 steps per minute. Gradually increase to twenty minutes a day at 80–90 steps per minute.

Running Start with one mile a day in eleven minutes (alternative running and walking) and gradually increase to two miles a day in seventeen minutes.

Swimming Start with one hundred yards a day in two and a half minutes, and gradually increase to one thousand yards a day at a rate of one hundred yards every two minutes.

Similarly, in other activities start with a level of exercise that is comfortably within your reach, and build up slowly to longer periods of more intense activity. The older you are, the more gently you should take it. If you start from complete inactivity, exercise yourself on alternate days for the first fortnight, then daily. Once you've achieved the level of fitness you want you can exercise on alternate days again.

Judging when you've had enough exercise is not easy. Considerable strain, but not too much, should be put on your muscles, heart and breathing. By the end of your routine, you should be panting but not having to gulp for breath. Your heart should be beating faster but not pounding uncomfortably. If in doubt about whether you are pushing yourself too fast (or too slowly), consult a physical education teacher, or even a doctor.

What are the different types of exercise, and what do they achieve?

Different types of exercise strengthen your body in different ways. Which kind you undertake will depend on what result you want to achieve.

Circulo-respiratory (CR) *exercises* improve your general fitness. This category includes nearly all active sports, and also walking, jogging, running and skipping and rowing and cycling machines.

Flexibility exercises involve stretching and rotating the body. They are recommended to overcome stiffness and muscular tension, and can also help to prevent arthritis. They include dance exercises and yoga.

Isometric exercises are designed to increase your ability to exert force against a fixed resistance. Samson exerted isometric strength, for instance, when he held the pillars of the temple apart. The exercises typically involve no movement at

17

all; instead you flex your muscles against a fixed object like a wall or a bar.

Isotonic exercises develop isotonic strength: the ability to exert force through the whole range of movement of a given joint. Weightlifting, which provides a continuous resistance to movement, is the archetypal isotonic routine.

Endurance exercises are designed to increase your ability to exert force for long periods of time. Traditional calisthenics, including push-ups, sit-ups and squat-leg-thrusts, are typical of such exercises.

Can exercise be harmful?

Moderate and regular exercise is the best way to get and stay fit, and can do you no harm. But the man who rushes out after weeks or years of inactivity and throws himself into sudden, unaccustomed exercise is asking for trouble, especially if he is over thirty-five years old. Your body is a delicate system, and an unfit body, like a new car, needs a period of "running in." A number of commonsense rules will avoid physical strain or injury.

First, always warm up before a bout of vigorous exercise, especially in cold weather. Sudden activity when you're cold can make your blood pressure soar. Sudden movements of stiff joints and muscles can lead to painful sprains and wrenches.

Secondly, slow down gradually after violent exercise; don't stop all at once.

Thirdly, when beginning a new sport or set of exercises, learn the movements gradually, so that your body can become accustomed to them without strain.

In other words, take it gently. Going out once a week and driving yourself till your heart pounds is not only stupid but also much less effective than short daily bouts of moderate exertion.

Sudden and inappropriate exercise can damage the heart or

other parts of the body. If you think you have a weak heart, or if you are over thirty-five years old and have been inactive for some time, it is a good idea to consult your doctor before taking up a sport or starting a regime of exercises. Careful and regular exercise, however, can strengthen even badly diseased hearts.

BODY ODORS

What causes body odor?

Your *body odor* (BO) is your own natural smell, and in earlier eras might have been perfectly acceptable. Nowadays, however, social convention requires you to replace your own smell with a manufactured one, usually expensive. The cosmetic conspiracy has taken over.

Body odor is caused by your sweat. Most perspiration is basically salt water and gives off little smell; but the perspiration from your armpits and crotch contains fatty substances which exude a rancid odor when they oxidize in the air. This kind of sweat also provides an ideal breeding ground for bacteria which are harmless except for the smell they produce. Up to 95 percent of your BO comes from your armpits, crotch and feet.

Both sweating and BO can be increased by obesity, spicy foods, coffee and some forms of alcohol.

What can I do about BO?

There are three stages of treatment. First, *wash daily*, especially your armpits, crotch and feet. If you suffer from bad BO, use a soap that contains a deodorant or anti-bacterial agent.

Secondly, *use a deodorant*. Most deodorants contain a bacteriostat, alcohol, perfume and sometimes a conditioning oil. They come in roll-on, spray-can cream, soap and other forms. Aerosol sprays are now believed to damage the

19

environment (by affecting the ozone layer in the atmosphere) so a roll-on is more suitable for the ecologically conscious.

Thirdly, *use an antiperspirant*. These reduce sweating by blocking the sweat pores. Many antiperspirants contain a deodorant, and vice versa. Again, they come in roll-on (or cream) as well as aerosol form. If you are worried that blocking your pores may be bad for you, don't. You have two to five million pores on your body, and applying an antiperspirant to your armpits and a few other selected areas is unlikely to impair your bodily functioning.

Problems that do arise are, first, that some people are allergic to deodorant or antiperspirant substances; secondly that your odor-producing bacteria may adapt and become resistant to the substance you use to kill them. Changing the brand may solve this problem – if the new brand contains different substances.

If I sweat a lot, does it mean there's something wrong?

Sweating is the primary means by which your body maintains a consistent internal temperature. When your body heats up – in the sun, when you exercise, or when you're feverish – the blood vessels in and near the skin dilate, and heat is radiated out. Sweat is produced in your pores. It is mostly salt water, with some chemicals, poisonous waste and fatty substances mixed in.

Most people sweat about half a pint a day, but this will vary enormously according to climate and activity. Sweating can also be increased by being overweight and by eating particular foods, such as hot curries.

If you're still convinced that you sweat an abnormal amount, consult a doctor.

What about foot odor?

Foot odor is due not so much to the kind of sweat that feet exude as to the confined conditions in which they are normally kept. Swaddled in socks and shoes, your feet are cut off from natural air conditioning. The sweat from your feet has no chance to evaporate and instead provides the ideal bacterial breeding ground. A few people suffer from abnormally offensive foot odor, a condition known as *bromidrosis*.

To treat foot odor, wash your feet – especially between the toes – once or twice a day. Use a foot deodorant or antiperspirant, or dust between your toes and inside your socks with anti-bacterial powder. Change your socks at least once a day. Change and thoroughly air your shoes regularly. Go barefoot or wear sandals whenever possible.

With bromidrosis, more extreme measures may also be necessary, including repeated bathing of the feet in hot and then cold water, and regular disinfection of socks and shoes.

What causes bad breath?

Bad breath (or *halitosis*) is caused by problems in your mouth or stomach, or both. Decaying teeth and infected gums are a major factor. So is failure to brush your teeth regularly to clean away accumulated plaque and food particles (see TEETH). Constipation, upset stomach and major changes in diet can also cause halitosis. A dry mouth at times of stress and tension turns the breath sour.

What can I do about bad breath?

The most effective treatment is to keep your mouth clean, by brushing your teeth, front and back, at least once a day, and preferably after each meal. If you've got tooth decay or gum disease, you should visit a dentist. A regular diet also helps.

Mouthwashes have only a temporary effect, and freshen your mouth without combating the cause of the problem.

Similarly, various chewing gums, sprays, tablets and candy can temporarily mask the problem.

SKIN

What exactly is skin?

Your skin is a double-layered, 1–4 millimeter thick sheet of body cells which covers an area of about twenty square feet and accounts for some 16 percent of your body weight. It is sensitive, elastic, oily and sweaty, and covers you from crown to toe.

The outer layer or *epidermis* consists of tightly packed, tough, dead cells which flake off naturally at a rate of about one gram per day and are replaced by new skin from the dermis below. The *dermis* itself is a complex environment which includes elastic fibers, blood vessels, nerve endings, hair follicles, sweat pores, and glands that produce oil, pigment and perspiration.

Your skin is colored genetically with varying quantities of a pigment called *melanin*. Albinos are people without melanin. You may range in color from pink to dark brown according to your race and the environment in which you live. The "tanning" of white people is caused by increased secretion of pigment due to excessive exposure to the sun.

As you grow older, the replacement of epidermis cells slows down, so that your outer skin tends to become scaly and cracked. Wrinkles appear as the dermis gradually shrinks and loses its elasticity.

What causes dry or oily skin?

The oiliness of your skin depends on the activity of your *sebaceous glands*, which produce a fatty substance called *sebum*. This lubricates both your skin and your hair. At puberty, male hormones increase the output of these glands, and it is the increased oiliness of the skin over the next few years that makes teenagers so liable to pimples and acne. As you grow older, the activity of the sebaceous glands declines.

Washing with soap removes not only dirt but also some of the oil from the skin. Too much washing, or washing with detergents, can lead to dryness of the skin and irritation.

How often should I wash? Is a shower more hygienic than a bath?

Washing is as much a cosmetic as a hygienic activity. The natural body odor produced by the sweat and oil on your skin is regarded as distasteful in modern societies, but there is nothing unhygienic about it. Many of the bacteria that live on human skin are there to protect you, not infect you. Indeed, it is possible that too much washing will remove natural forms of protection and make your skin more liable to infection or other problems.

Given all that, regular washing both cleans you and makes you socially acceptable. Depending on your type of work, you should need to wash only once a day. More frequent washing can help very oily skin, but may harm dry skin.

Showers use a great deal less water than baths – an important factor in many parts of the world – but they are not noticeably more hygienic. Some people seem to think that having a bath involves wallowing in your own dirt; others regard a good hot bath as one of the pleasures of life.

Is sunbathing good or bad for the skin?

Not much more than one hundred years ago bronzed skin was associated with menial outdoor work and regarded as a sign of inferior class. Fashionable ladies used to pride themselves on the milky whiteness of their bodies, and used parasols to protect their faces from the sun's rays. But now that most working-class people toil away in factories and have skins whiter than snow, a suntan is regarded as the epitome of fashion, indicating that you have the wealth to laze about on beaches and ski runs.

The medical fact, however, is that excessive sunbathing is bad for you. There is some evidence that consistent exposure to the sun's ultraviolet radiation increases your chances of getting skin cancer. If noticed early, skin cancers are quite easily dealt with. But if neglected, they can spread beneath the skin and to other parts of the body.

The bronzing of your skin by sunbathing is due to increased production of melanin pigment, a natural defense mechanism to protect you from solar ultraviolet rays. Skin that is tanned regularly tends to age prematurely, becoming dry, inelastic, leathery and wrinkled.

Fair-skinned people are in constant danger of sunburn.

What is sunburn?

People who have a low melanin content in their skins are liable to be sunburnt after overexposure to the sun. In most cases, sunburn is similar to superficial heat burns, though it may be several hours before you notice it. The skin turns red, itchy, and painful to the touch; a day or two later it may peel off. Mild sunburn can be treated with a number of over-the-counter lotions. In severe cases, hospital treatment may be necessary. Fair-skinned people should build up their tolerance to the sun's rays by frequent brief periods of exposure. This gradually increases the melanin content in the skin. Suntan lotions also help.

What causes blackheads and whiteheads? What can I do about them?

Blackheads and whiteheads occur either as a result of over-production of sebum or because pores are blocked by dirt or dust. The result is a wax-like plug known as a *comedo*. If it is open to the air, the end of the comedo turns black and forms a blackhead; if covered by skin, the result is a whitehead.

To remove a pimple, first open the pores by washing your face in warm water – otherwise the pore may remain open after the blackhead has been removed. Next, squeeze the pimple out gently. Rough treatment is likely to damage and inflame the surrounding skin and spread infection. Finally, after removing the pimple, wash thoroughly with antiseptic soap.

To avoid pimples, you should wash your face thoroughly at least once a day, avoid greasy foods or cosmetics, and get plenty of fresh air.

Is it possible to cure acne?

Acne is an extremely intractable condition common among teenagers. It appears to be caused by stimulation of the skin by the male sex hormones following puberty, and is related to the increased production of oil by the sebaceous glands. The result is pimples or pustules that swell up on the face, neck, chest and back. These produce pus, and leave scars for some time afterward.

Though various lotions, frequent washing, exposure to sunlight and avoidance of greasy foods can help, they will neither prevent nor cure acne. The only certain cure is time. But if your condition is severe, consult your doctor.

What should I do about a boil?

Boils are large pustules which develop in hair follicles or sweat pores. They typically swell up painfully over a period of several days. Sometimes they subside of their own accord. If they neither subside nor discharge by themselves, they should be lanced by a doctor. Squeezing a boil or do-it-yourself lancing is liable to spread the problem or lead to infection of the wound and possible blood poisoning. If the boil discharges itself, you should clean the area thoroughly, and apply an antiseptic and a dressing.

Boils sometimes come several at a time, or one after another. If so, you should consult a doctor, as there may be some underlying condition that is causing the trouble.

What is dermatitis?

Dermatitis and *eczema* both describe a number of ill-defined conditions that produce inflammation of the skin. They often involve some kind of allergy produced either by exposure to an irritant substance, or by some psychosomatic mechanism. Physical causes of dermatitis include cosmetics, foods, dyes, chemicals, fabrics, paints, detergents, plastics, even rubber and metals. Contact with the offending substance leads to a rash and blisters which eventually rupture and form sores. The skin thickens, and flakes off in scales.

The only certain cure in such cases is to find out what substance is affecting you and avoid it. If it is something you come into contact with at work, consult your own or the company doctor; you may need to wear protective clothing or to have special washing facilities.

If the condition is psychosomatic, a cure is more difficult to find. Consult a doctor.

What are hives?

They are painful red areas of swollen skin that can range in size from a coin to a plate. They are caused by dust or pollen, an allergic reaction or emotional stress.

Hives are unpleasant but not serious. As with dermatitis,

the means of cure usually lies in identifying and avoiding the causative substance. The hives themselves can be alleviated with soothing lotions – consult a pharmacist or doctor. Allergy-based hives may be treated with antihistamines.

How can I get rid of warts?

Warts and *plantar warts* (which appear on the soles of the feet) are viral infections which usually go away of their own accord within three to twenty-four months. But if you can't wait that long, or if a plantar wart makes walking painful, they can also be removed by physical means: they can be cut out, or removed by freezing or corrosive fluids. Consult a doctor for treatment.

HAIR

What are the different types of hair?

Hairs are tubes of proteins which grow from roots (or follicles) embedded in your skin. They cover the whole of your body except the palms of your hands, the soles of your feet, and parts of your genitals. Three types of hair are usually distinguished – body hair, sexual hair, and scalp hair.

Body hair tends to be shorter and less pigmented than sexual or scalp hair. It is a sign of mankind's steady evolution toward baldness – not that we have fewer hairs, but shorter ones. Both men and women, in fact, have a similar number of follicles to gorillas, but most of these hairs are so fine and small as to be invisible.

Sexual hair includes not only pubic hair but also the hair on your chest, your armpits, and your face. Its growth is dependent on male sex hormones, which is why your beard hair continues to grow even when your scalp is becoming bald.

The growth of *scalp hair* is dependent on another hormone,

androgen. The normal rate of growth is about a third of a millimeter a day, and occurs over a cycle lasting about three years. At the end of the growth cycle, the hair is expelled from the follicle – which is why it is perfectly natural for you to shed some fifty to one hundred hairs each day. The follicle then rests for a period of about three months before beginning to manufacture a new hair. Most men have about 1,000 hairs per square inch of scalp, and about 120,000 scalp hairs in all.

Is it true that hair grows faster, or becomes coarser, the more often it's cut or shaved?

This is a myth. Hair on your face or your scalp (or any part of your body) grows at much the same rate however frequently you shave or visit the hairdresser. On the other hand, both the rate of growth and the quality and luster of your hair are affected by such things as extreme dietary deficiencies or changes, physical illness, anxiety and stress, and a number of scalp conditions, including dandruff and skin infections.

How is hair colored? What makes it go gray?

Like skin color, hair color is determined genetically. It is the result of the type and quantity of pigment put into the protein when each hair is being manufactured. As you grow older, your follicles tend to produce less pigment, and the hairs become colorless. Hair does not *turn* gray. Gray hair is the product of a mixture of colored and colorless hairs. When all your pigmented hairs have been shed, and no more are being produced, the result is white hair.

The tendency to go gray seems to be inherited. Some men's hair becomes gray sooner than others'. A common myth is that sudden shock or grief can turn your hair gray. This is not so. What seems to happen is that under extreme stress your scalp sheds older, colored hairs at a faster than usual rate, so that your hair may appear to go gray quite suddenly.

Once your body has ceased producing hair pigment, there is no known way to revive or stimulate it. Either you make the best of your gray hair – and it can look very handsome – or you resort to dyes.

What can I do about dry or oily hair?

Each hair follicle contains a sebaceous gland which secretes an oily substance to lubricate and protect your hair. The activity of these glands determines how dry or oily your hair is.

Shampoos and hair conditioners are usually made for dry, normal and oily hair. If you choose one suited to your type of hair, you should be able to avoid excessive dryness or oiliness. If you have doubts, consult your hairdresser.

How often should I wash my hair?

As often as you need to keep it clean. In polluted cities, this may be every day. Water doesn't damage your hair, and washing it as often as three times a day will not hurt it. In an unpolluted environment, most hairdressers advise washing every two days if you have oily hair, every four to five days if you have dry hair.

Use a shampoo. Ordinary soap tends to dry the hair out and leave a dull film on it. As for which shampoo to use, that depends on the type and condition of your hair, and on whether a particular product seems to work for you. If it doesn't, try another. Read the labels. Ignore TV ads and gimmicks, and don't assume that the more expensive the shampoo the better it will be.

Should I use a brush or a comb?

Some "experts" claim brushes are wicked, but others disagree.

It's largely a matter of fashion. Whether you use brush or comb, keep it clean to avoid spreading bacteria and infection, and apply gently, especially when your hair is wet and vulnerable to splitting and stretching. Do not back-comb, as this strips the protective layer off the hairs. Do not use a comb whose teeth are sharp, for the same reason.

Does scalp massage help my hair?

It's a common belief that scalp massage contributes to the health and growth of your hair by stimulating the supply of blood and nutrients to the follicles. It may also induce a sense of relaxation and well-being. There is no evidence, however, that regularly massaging your scalp will either prevent or retard baldness or grayness.

If you do massage your scalp, don't let your fingers massage your hair instead, since this can damage it. Get a firm grip on the skin and move it to and fro; don't rub.

What causes dandruff? What can I do about it?

Dandruff is a harmless but unsightly condition whose precise cause remains unknown. There are two types: fine, dry scales which fall from the scalp and tend to bedeck your shoulders; and thick, greasy scales which stay on the scalp.

If you suffer from dandruff, the first step is to try the various medicated shampoos on the market. Some contain little more than simple antiseptics, while others are a mixture of strong chemicals. Follow the instructions and use for at least two weeks; if it doesn't work, try another. If nothing seems to work, consult a doctor as the dandruff may be the result of some skin disorder.

What can I do about hair lice?

The hair louse (*Pediculus humanus*) is an itchy and tenacious beast which can be acquired not only from infected people but also from hats, brushes and combs. The lice themselves tend to stay well hidden but their eggs or "nits" can be seen attached to the hair shafts near their roots. Head lice are difficult to kill, and simple washing, even in very hot water, won't work. Consult a doctor or pharmacist; a special type of shampoo will be in order, and perhaps other treatment.

What causes baldness?

Thinning of the hair and eventual baldness occur when the follicles on your scalp stop producing normal full-length hairs. This isn't necessarily because the follicles are dead; most often they continue to produce, but the result is a delicate fuzz similar to very fine body hair.

A degree of thinning of the hair is common to both men and women as they grow older, but baldness is particularly a male phenomenon. No one knows just what causes it, and there is no known means of preventing or curing it. Baldness does, however, seem to be inherited. If your father or grandfathers went bald, the chances are you will follow suit. Mental and emotional stress are also said to be contributory factors, but since many men who suffer from stress nonetheless retain a full head of hair, its role remains uncertain.

Hair loss can also be caused by burns or other injuries that destroy the hair follicles; by certain skin diseases such as *dermatitis* and *psoriasis*; by some other diseases, such as *anemia*; and by various forms of pollution, including mercury and radiation poisoning.

Men's magazines usually carry advertisements for a number of wild and expensive treatments guaranteed to prevent or cure baldness. No doubt some of them do work occasionally, but be warned: there is *no* guarantee, and the chances are that you will just go on getting bald.

Is baldness a sign of impotence? Or of virility?

In spite of Samson's problems with Delilah, there's no evidence that the amount or length of hair on your head has anything to do with your sexual desire or potency. Of course, if you're utterly convinced that your abilities with women are connected with your hair, baldness may well cause a psychological reaction. But you can reassure yourself with the apparent virility of such well-known baldies as Yul Brynner and Telly Savalas.

The idea that baldness actually increases virility seems to have been deduced from the fact that eunuchs never go bald. Logically, however, it doesn't follow that bald men never become "eunuchs." Some bald men may of course have an extra need, because of their shiny scalp, to prove to themselves that they can still be attractive to women.

Will baldness make me less attractive?

Beauty is in the eye (or ear, or mind) of the beholder. Baldness need not be the awful disability that so many men believe it to be. Bald can be beautiful. It's largely a question of self-confidence. There are many women who find bald or balding men extremely attractive.

What often is unattractive – because of the vanity, insecurity and dishonesty it reveals – is the desperate attempt many men make to conceal loss of hair. The moment you finally reveal to your partner that your hair is, in fact, false can be embarrassing and undignified.

I've heard about hair weaving and hair transplants. What are they and do they work?

There are two types of *hair weaving*. In the first, an ordinary hairpiece is attached to the scalp by stitching its edges to your own hair. In the second, a grid of threads is strung across the bald patch and "wefts" or wedges of hair are sewn directly onto it. The problem with both types is that as your own hair continues to grow, the woven hair becomes increasingly loose. So you have to go back for a refit about every six weeks, which makes the whole thing an expensive process. The constant pulling of the hairweave on your own hair may also accelerate hair loss.

Hair transplantation is a surgical process in which a group or "plug" of follicles is removed from a part of your head where the hair is growing normally (usually the nape of the neck) and reinserted in a balding area. The shock of the transplant causes the existing hairs in the plug to fall out, and it will be some months before new ones start to grow. Each plug contains twelve to eighteen roots, of which only six to fourteen may sprout successfully. It will therefore be up to six months before you know how successful the transplant has been. In some cases, for reasons that are unclear, the transplant doesn't "take" at all.

Transplants are relatively expensive, but on the whole they do appear to be a successful answer to baldness. But we cannot be certain yet because the technique is still quite recent, so no one knows whether transplanted hair will continue growing after ten or twenty years.

The actual surgery is messy, because of all the blood vessels in the scalp, but not particularly painful. About 150 plugs can be transplanted at a single session. The head is then swathed in bandages for up to a week, and remains covered with congealed blood until the scabs fall off naturally.

One problem with transplantation is that your normal hair will continue to disappear, so that you may require further transplants to keep up appearances. Quite apart from the cost and inconvenience, you must consider whether you're not fighting a battle that you are bound to lose in the end.

What about hairpieces and wigs?

Hairpieces (*toupees*) and *wigs* are the traditional means of covering up hair loss, but they have a number of disadvantages you should consider before deciding to hide your baldness. First, they are expensive – a good piece (and a bad one is worse than none at all) costs up to $400, a good wig up to $600. Secondly, they require a great deal of washing, styling and other maintenance. Thirdly, there's a problem in matching the color of a hairpiece to your own hair; even if you get a good match to start with, your own hair will gradually change in color. Fourthly, it's a bad idea to keep your wig or hairpiece on at times when you may feel most in need of it – when swimming, playing rough sports, and in bed. Lastly, you are, in effect, committing a deception which your intimate (and not so intimate) acquaintances are bound to discover sooner or later; accidental revelation of the real state of your hair can be acutely embarrassing.

Whether these difficulties are outweighed by the more youthful appearance and sense of self-confidence that a person gains from not appearing bald can only be decided by each individual. But baldness is not a calamity. Though people may tease you about it, it won't disfigure or incapacitate you.

How often do men usually need to shave?

It all depends on how concerned you are to remain clean-shaven. Most men shave once a day. If your hair is dark, producing a five o'clock shadow, you may want to shave morning and evening.

Is wet or dry shaving better?

As long as you are shaven, it makes very little difference which method you use. Electric razors leave beard hairs with ragged instead of clean-cut ends, but the difference is only visible under a powerful microscope. Whichever method you find most effective and convenient is the best.

EYES

How can I tell if I need eyeglasses?

If you have difficulty in focusing sharply, either in general or on objects that are close up or far away, you should consult an oculist or optometrist to see whether you need spectacles (or contact lenses). (Optometrists test your sight, oculists treat eye defects.) Eyeglasses are prescribed for three main conditions:

Near-sightedness (myopia) means that you have difficulty in focusing on distant objects, which appear blurred. Concave lenses are needed to correct the problem.

Far-sightedness (hypermetropia) is the opposite, and means you have difficulty in focusing on objects close to you. The condition often leads to eye-strain and headaches, especially after a prolonged period of close visual activity such as reading. Convex lenses solve the problem.

Astigmatism means that you have difficulty in focusing on vertical and horizontal lines simultaneously. Typically, part of an object will be in sharp focus while another part is blurred. Vision may be generally distorted, circles appearing as ovals and square shapes appearing to be elongated. Points of light may appear to have trails. A special type of lens is required for this condition.

Another problem that occurs in middle and old age is *presbyopia*, in which a hardening of the lens of the eye makes it increasingly difficult to adjust focus and especially to focus on objects close at hand. As with far-sightedness, convex lenses are needed.

Eyeglasses or contact lenses?

Many people whose eyesight is defective prefer contact lenses because they think eyeglasses will destroy their looks, or age them overnight. Chosen carefully, however, eyeglasses can suit a man and enhance his appearance. They can also be useful props. Contact lenses, on the other hand, are necessary if you lead a particularly active life. Apart from such questions, there's little to choose between the two.

Contact lenses are small, wafer-thin disks of splinter-proof plastic which are chosen to suit the curve of your eye (there are about fifty-six varieties of eye curve). It takes some three to four weeks for your eyes to get accustomed to the lenses, but after this breaking-in period you may well forget you are wearing them. Problems arise if your lenses fall out: they are difficult to find and easily damaged.

Contact lenses come in two types: hard and soft. Hard lenses float on a film of tear fluid and can either cover the whole visible area of the eye (*scleral lenses*) or just the center of the eye *(corneal lenses)*. Scleral lenses are recommended for people who indulge in strenuous sports since they are least likely to fall out. Soft lenses differ from hard ones in that they absorb water from the tear fluid, which makes them more immediately comfortable. They can also be left off for several days, and then worn again without discomfort. Hard lenses, however, are less easily damaged, cheaper, and longer-lasting (six to eight years as compared to two to three years for soft lenses). Both types need to be cleaned regularly and kept in a special fluid when out of the eyes.

What causes color blindness?

Normal eyes contain nerve-endings to distinguish three primary colors: red, green and blue. By far the most common form of *color blindness* is an absence of nerve-endings that recognize red. The result is an inability to distinguish between red and green. 8 percent of men and 0.4 percent of women have this difficulty. The inequality between the sexes is due to the defect being a sex-linked genetic characteristic: a woman can transmit it to her son without herself being affected. Women only have the defect if they have both a color-blind father and a "carrier" mother.

Color blindness is a minor disability except in certain jobs where the recognition of red and green is important, for instance on the railroads or at sea. There is no known cure.

TEETH

What causes tooth decay?

Tooth decay is the single most common physical problem in modern societies. In Britain, one third of all adults are completely toothless and wear a full set of dentures. And Americans aren't far behind.

The decay starts when certain bacteria (*lactobacilli*) convert sugar in the food you eat into acid. This acid eats through the enamel covering of the teeth and forms cavities where the bacteria can really get to work. Your mouth is full of bacteria, and most of them are harmless. Lactobacilli are also harmless as long as they are exposed to the air; this exposure is the most important function of brushing your teeth. When you don't brush regularly, however, a film of protein, bacteria and food particles known as "plaque" covers the teeth and allows the bacteria to eat away at the enamel.

Sweet foods are the main cause of tooth decay. Failure to brush the teeth after meals compounds the problem.

How can I prevent tooth decay?

The most important factor is a well-balanced diet that avoids an excess of sugar and starch. The second most important factor is brushing your teeth after every meal and snack. When sugar was rationed in Britain during World War II, the number of cavities among children fell dramatically.

If decay has already started, you should immediately visit a dentist. Just because decay is painless, at least initially, doesn't mean that it's not at work. If you let it continue, you'll end up another denture statistic.

What about fluoride?

Fluoride is a chemical which helps to reduce tooth decay by hardening the enamel, but it only benefits the teeth of children under the age of fourteen. Small amounts of fluoride may be put in the public water supply, or in toothpaste. In the US, fluoride is given to children on a regular basis.

Are some kinds of toothpaste better than others?
Is there a preferred method of brushing the teeth?

Toothpaste that contains fluoride benefits children, but apart from this there is nothing to suggest that one brand of toothpaste is any better at fighting tooth decay than another. Indeed, brushing your teeth with plain salt is not only cheap and good for the gums, but also cleans the teeth just as effectively as paste. Nor is it true that toothpaste will make your teeth whiter than white. Most people's teeth are naturally slightly yellow, and they tend to get slightly more yellow as you grow older. Smoking, however, may stain the teeth unnaturally.

As for brushing, the most important thing is simply to get your teeth clean, front, back and in-between. The method you use to achieve this is of secondary importance, and the recommended action seems to change every few years. A useful device, available from pharmacists in the US and dentists in Britain is a stain tablet which colors plaque red. Taken after you've brushed your teeth, it will show clearly how effective your technique is and which areas to concentrate on in future.

What about gum disease?

Periodontal or *gum diseases* attack the supporting structures of your teeth and, if untreated, can lead to loosening and eventually loss of teeth. The most common problem is where the gum tends to become soft and detached from the teeth. This enlarges the socket of the tooth and destroys the securing fibers that hold it in place. It can lead to painful abscesses in the gums. If you have this or any other gum problem, you should consult a dentist.

Causes of gum disease are much the same as the causes of tooth decay: sweet and soft foods, insufficient or inefficient brushing, deposits of food particles, irregular teeth, and also badly fitting dentures.

FEET

What can I do about flat feet?

Flat feet are a common ailment, the seriousness of which has been largely exaggerated. Flat feet are not a deformity and many people, including some top athletes, manage perfectly well in spite of them. The aches and pains associated with flat feet are usually due to the process by which they become flat – falling arches – rather than to the flatness itself.

Your feet are each equipped with three and a half arches. Two run from your toes to your heels, another runs across the joints of your toes, and the half arch runs across the middle of the foot. The result is the typical footprint with its narrow "waist" between toes and heel. Feet become flat when one or more of these arches weakens and falls.

Falling arches can be caused by badly fitting shoes, weak feet and leg muscles, poor posture, overweight, regularly carrying heavy loads or standing still for long periods, and by injuries and arthritis. Whatever the cause of the strain, the muscles and ligaments that hold your arches up prove insufficient to carry the load; the arches begin to collapse, causing pain and fatigue in your legs and feet.

If you suffer from this problem, you should consult a chiropodist (foot expert) or a doctor. There are several possible treatments, including shoes with built-in arch supports and exercises to strengthen your foot and leg muscles. If caught in time, falling arches can be corrected.

What should I look for when I choose a pair of shoes?

Most of us buy shoes for their looks rather than their comfort: a habit that can lead to problems as various as blisters, foot odor, corns, calluses and flat feet.

Your feet have to support the entire weight of your body, and should be treated with appropriate respect.

Good shoes give support to your feet and ankles without strain or friction. They fit tightly all around the heels so that they do not slip and rub when you walk. They allow room for your toes to move up and down and sideways. They bend at the same place that your foot bends, which avoids the agonizing process of forcing the shoes to adjust to your feet. They give firm support to your arches. And they are made of a material, like leather, which "breathes" easily, so that the circulation of air will reduce or eliminate foot odor. (Some plastic and synthetic materials also "breathe," but not as well as leather).

High heels tend to put undue strain on foot and leg muscles, and are therefore not recommended from the strictly physical point of view. The benefits of added height and style must be balanced against possible discomfort.

What can I do about ingrown toenails?

Ingrown toenails occur when the nails curl inward and grow into the skin. It is an unsightly and occasionally painful problem, which most frequently afflicts the big toes. To prevent ingrowing, nails should be cut *square* (not in a curve), so that the edges of the nail extend out from the skin. Tight shoes which press down on the nails are another cause of ingrowing.

If you already have ingrown nails, you could try the cure advocated by Russell L. Rhodes in his *Man at His Best* (Doubleday, 1974): wedge thin rolls of lamb's wool soaked in natural oil (e.g. olive oil) between the side grooves of the flesh and the ingrowing nail. This, he claims, will make the nail grow out again.

If this fails, consult a chiropodist.

What is athlete's foot?

Athlete's foot is a form of ringworm, a fungal infection of the outer layer of the skin. Its only association with athletes is that school and sports club changing rooms are likely locations for infection. In fact, even the most sedentary of men can fall victim to the complaint.

Athlete's foot first appears in the clefts between your toes, causing itching, splitting of the infected skin and the flaking of dead skin. If untreated, it may spread over the rest of your feet, and even to other parts of the body (legs, hands, groin).

Because the fungus thrives in dark and sweaty conditions, use of a foot powder in your socks and exposure of your feet to the air are major elements in the treatment. There are also a considerable number of over-the-counter creams and ointments which will supposedly kill the fungus and dry the infected area. If self-treatment with these remedies does not work, consult a chiropodist or doctor.

What's the difference between calluses and corns? What can I do about them?

Calluses are areas of hardened skin which result from continued friction and pressure (typically caused by ill-fitting shoes). Unless they become acute and press on nerve endings, they do not cause any trouble. They can be removed by abrasion with a pumice stone or an emery board or by a chiropodist – but such treatment will be futile unless the original cause of the friction and pressure is also removed.

Corns are smaller and more intense calluses. The hardening of the skin has a well-defined core which grows into your foot and presses painfully on nerve endings. Corns should be removed by a chiropodist. Corn plasters and pads usually provide only temporary relief by spreading the offending pressure over a wider area. Again, the cause of this pressure must be removed as well as the corn itself.

Sex

The "secret" of lovemaking, and the only rule about sex which is worth anything, is to understand what turns each other on.

In Masters and Johnson's classic phrase, "It takes two to make a sex problem." If your partners cannot bring themselves to tell you what they like, it is up to you to find out. And this cuts both ways, because an inability to express your own sexual needs is a form of illiteracy which leaves you ignorant of your own body and limits your relations with other people.

It is not always easy, but if you are too embarrassed to talk about sex openly, there are many ways of dropping hints, expressing degrees of pleasure while it is happening or joking about it afterward, which say all that is needed.

SEX ORGANS

What are the male sexual organs?

Most men assume that their sexual organs consist of a penis and two testicles, but there is much more to it than that – most of it is inside you. The female organs are elaborate, but they don't compare with the complexity of plumbing inside a man's body, which contains more than 8 feet of tubing with numerous valves, pumps and mixing chambers.

The *testes* are two flattened oval balls about $1\frac{3}{4}$ inches long and 1 inch wide, containing 2 or 3 feet of fine tubing, packed in like spaghetti. It is inside these tubes (*seminiferous tubules*) that the sperm are generated. Hundreds of thousands of independent organisms are produced in your testicles every hour of every day, each one of which carries a copy of your complete genetic code. The testes also manufacture the male sex hormone, *testosterone*, which is responsible for many masculine characteristics and, together with psychological factors, controls your sex drive. The testes are so efficient at maintaining the right level of testosterone in your body that if one of them is surgically removed, the other can make up the supply by itself.

In order to produce fertile sperm, the testes have to be kept a degree or two below body heat, which is why they hang outside the abdomen in your *scrotum*. This consists of two bags of skin joined together with a partition between, which controls the temperature by expanding to cool down or shrinking up against the body to warm up. Just beside the testes in each half of the scrotum are loose soft organs (the *epididymes*) in which the young sperm mature. When they are are fully grown, they move up from the testes into the body along two tubes called the *vas deferens*. These are about 16 inches long, curving up from the groin on either side and coming together to join the *urethra* just below the bladder.

The urethra is the main tube running down from the bladder and out through the penis, along which all your urine and semen passes.

Although it is buried deep inside you, the junction of the vas deferens and the urethra is a very sensitive and vulnerable part of your anatomy. It is wrapped around with an organ called the *prostate* – a complicated set of glands and muscles which, among other things, stores the sperm, produces seminal fluid and controls the muscles which allow you to urinate or ejaculate. The prostate is described in greater detail later, because it is the sex organ most likely to cause you medical problems.

The urethra is about 8 inches long and roughly S-shaped. It descends vertically from the prostate to a point between your legs, where you can feel it under a fold of skin called the *perineum* just behind the testicles. It then runs forward and slightly upward, through the back of the scrotum to the base of the penis.

The penis consists mainly of two strips of spongy tissue, side by side, with the urethra running underneath them to form a triangular cross-section, bound together by sheets of thin membrane. The head of the penis is called the *glans,* after the Latin for "acorn," and is usually the most sensitive part with a very high concentration of nerve endings. This is especially so on the underside, where a small flange of skin called the *frenum* joins the glans to the shaft. Unless this has been removed by circumcision, the glans is partly or wholly covered by a fold of skin called the foreskin, or *prepuce.*

The penis is a very individual part of the anatomy. It can come in a variety of shapes, sizes and colors – cylindrical, tapering, curved, thin or bulbous, long or short – as distinctive to a person as his face or fingerprint.

How did our sexual organs come to be where they are?

The shape and position of the human sexual organs are a compromise which evolved when our prototype ancestors first started to stand on their hind legs. Straightening up and walking upright meant that the rear-entry position for sexual intercourse, common to most of the animal kingdom, was abandoned in favor of a face-to-face position. The male organs became looser and hung vertically down, giving man the largest penis for his size of any mammal, and the woman's vagina "moved" forward as far as the ridge of the pubic bone would allow.

What are the main female sex organs?

During the first couple of months of pregnancy, it is difficult to distinguish the sex of a child, because we all start out with the same basic equipment, including two sex glands and a rudimentary opening in the lower abdomen. By the eleventh week the skin around the opening has either joined up to form a penis or folded back as a vagina, but it is not until the thirty-fourth week that the glands finally become sperm-producing testes or egg-producing ovaries.

The woman's *ovaries*, unlike the testes, remain within her body, and instead of feeding sperm up to the penis, they supply eggs down tubes (the *Fallopian tubes*) into the *uterus*, or womb. This is the chamber in which the sperm eventually fertilizes the egg and the fetus grows. The floor of the uterus has an opening in a wall of muscle called the *cervix* which leads down into the vagina below. The *vagina* is a muscular passage which is normally about 5 inches long but capable of considerable distension. It is usually moist, and this increases with sexual excitement and at certain times during the sexual cycle, to act as both natural lubricant and self-cleansing system.

The opening to the vagina is fairly complicated and probably best described from the outside in. The outer folds, which normally cover the vaginal opening like a pair of lips, are called the *labia majora* and are roughly similar to the skin of your scrotum, though more fleshy. When these are parted the inner lips, or *labia minora*, are visible. These are hairless, smooth and sensitive to touch. When the women is sexually aroused they usually swell up and darken in color.

The top or forward end of the labia minora form a little hood like a foreskin over the *clitoris*. This is an organ resembling a miniature penis, which is made of the same erectile tissue and is just as sensitive, although it does not have an opening at the tip. When a clitoris is erect and hard it can be any size from a tiny button to an inch or longer.

Below this, just inside the labia minora, is the opening of the urethra through which the woman urinates; and below this, in turn, is the deep opening into the vagina itself.

During childhood, the entrance is partly covered by a membrane of skin called the *hymen* or maidenhead. Although it is the traditional symbol of virginity, an "intact" hymen rarely covers the whole opening and, anyway, it can easily be stretched or split without involving sexual activity. In an adult, once the hymen has been broken, the edges remain to form small irregular-shaped folds of skin around the opening to the vaginal passage.

I'm worried that I have a small penis. What is the "average" size?

The size of your penis will not affect your sexual enjoyment, but worrying about it certainly will. Your anxiety or embarrassment can easily communicate itself to your partner and her response will only reinforce your worry. It is far better to accept that everyone's body is different, and learn to enjoy the one you have.

Variations in recorded penis length range from over 12 inches to a fully operational erection only $\frac{1}{2}$ inch long. If such figures have any meaning, the "average" is about 3.75 inches (flaccid) and just over 6 inches (erect). The size of the penis bears less relationship to body size than any other organ, and the flaccid size gives no indication of how much it will enlarge on erection. Body type as opposed to body size does make a slight difference – ectomorphs (tall thin people) average 6.3 inches whereas endomorphs (stocky people) only average 6 inches – but there are no other indicators. Contrary to popular belief the penis bears no relationship to the size of the feet, the length of the nose or any other external sign.

If you are worried about the size of your penis, remember that it is not a mechanical instrument but a means of *receiving* sensations. It is how it *feels* that matters.

Is there any way to increase the size of my penis?

There are devices on the market, based on the principle of vacuum pumps, that claim to increase the size of your penis by regular "exercise." There is no evidence that they work, because it is a remarkably elastic organ and stretching will have little effect on its permanent length once it has reached adult size.

How important is penis size to a woman? I've read that technique in lovemaking is what really matters – but surely size does too?

The length of a penis often becomes a status symbol for a man, and some women share this belief, but it makes relatively little difference to their physical satisfaction. Since the most sensitive areas are around the opening to a woman's vagina, the depth of penetration is less important than manipulative techniques. The stimulation of the clitoris does not depend on penis size, and the vagina itself can adjust to accommodate any shape. What really matters is not size or technique, but whatever enables you to discover or invent ways of love-making that are fulfilling to both of you.

It is probably true to say that penis size is as important to women as breast size is to men. Some people are specifically turned on by the "well hung" or the "well stacked," but no woman is really disappointed if her partner is average.

It *is* sometimes physically possible for you to be too small (or too big), for you or your partner to come to orgasm in some positions. If you are worried about it, you might say, quite simply, "I know it's small, show me how it is best for you," and discover that your partner had sensed your concern and wanted to reassure you. Having talked about it, you could openly explore techniques of lovemaking and learn to respond to each other's needs. You might even stop worrying about penis size.

What are the advantages and disadvantages of circumcision? For instance, which do women prefer – circumcised or uncircumcised penises?

Circumcision, or cutting off the foreskin from around the head of the penis, is a social or religious operation rather than a medical one. There is no evidence that it makes any difference to sexual sensitivity or the time it takes to reach arousal or orgasm – though there are a number of popular myths about the subject.

In some cases circumcision is necessary because the foreskin is painfully tight, but the only real argument for the operation concerns a greasy deposit called *smegma*, which tends to collect under the foreskin. If not washed regularly it can smell unpleasantly and make the skin inflamed. More seriously, recent research has shown a connection between smegma and cancer in both men and women. However, normal hygiene deals with the problem, and many opponents of the operation consider it an unnecessary and unsightly mutilation. But many cultures take the opposite view. Male Jews and Moslems are circumcised as a religious requirement, and it is common practice in some Western countries.

Women vary as much as men in their opinions. During lovemaking, some prefer the additional folds of skin to manipulate, while others prefer the exposed shape of the glans. It usually comes down to an aesthetic judgment. If a woman likes you, she won't complain, provided that you are happy with (or without) it.

Can circumcision be performed on an adult?

Circumcision is often performed on adults, but it is a more complicated business which takes longer to heal than the simple operation carried out on a child. For instance, you will have to avoid having an erection for several weeks, and accidental sexual excitement could have painful results. As a rule, the adult operation only takes place for reasons of medical necessity or religious conversion.

Is it a reversible operation?

When there are strong psychological reasons for it, the foreskin can be replaced, using skin and tissue from other parts of your body, as a form of cosmetic surgery.

Is there a female equivalent to circumcision?

Female circumcision covers a wide range of operations, from removing the foreskin of the clitoris (the equivalent of the male operation) to removing the entire vulva leaving nothing but a massive scar. These monstrous and totally unnecessary practises are usually carried out in the name of religion. Fortunately they are now almost unknown in the West, but still take place in many parts of the world.

What happens when one's testicles drop at puberty?

The testes develop in the abdomen and usually descend into the scrotum about a month before birth. If they get stuck and remain in the body, the condition (called *cryptorchism*) may need to be corrected surgically, but it is common for them to descend naturally during childhood and before puberty. Testes which remain in the abdomen at puberty become infertile.

In the early years the scrotum tends to be tight against the body, but when the testes become operational and start producing sperm, they enlarge and the whole scrotum loosens up to give them room. This is the process that boys notice about themselves at puberty, and what they usually mean when they refer to the testicles "dropping."

I've heard that some people only have one testicle, or none at all. Can such people still have children?

It is possible for one testicle to descend but not the other. This does not interfere with sexual activity or fertility, provided that the descended testicle is in working order. It simply takes over the job of two.

When neither testicle has descended, the person is infertile, although he can still enjoy orgasm and produce semen.

Why does one testicle hang higher than the other?

About the only part of your body which is outwardly asymmetrical is the scrotum. The left testicle is usually lower than the right and has a slightly larger scrotal sac. This arrangement originally evolved so that they could hang more comfortably between the legs. In most other animals, the testicles project behind and are parallel.

What makes the scrotum tighten up or hang loose?

When you are relaxed, the scrotum hangs in loose folds to expose the maximum skin area and keep the testicles cool. But if it is too cold, or your hormone system responds to stress or sexual excitement, your muscles will contract, the testicles will be raised and the scrotum will be pulled into a tight shape against your body.

Does pubic hair serve any useful function?

Once, a very long time ago, body hair had a purpose. When we were primitive animals it was a practical insulation against heat and cold. It also protected the skin from knocks and abrasions, and provided a useful screen to protect the orifices from intrusion by insects. However, except for the hair on your head which still offers considerable protection, these defences no longer apply. In fact, we are steadily evolving toward a hairless condition, and the pubic hair growth just happens to be the last to go. Pubic hair also helps to retain our sexual smells, once very important for breeding, which is why the hormones promote additional growth at puberty.

Why is pubic hair crinkly, when the hair on my head is straight?

Pubic hair is a flattened oval shape in cross-section, which produces short, highly curled and wiry growth. It is tough and resilient and makes an ideal buffer to protect sensitive areas of the body. The main purpose of the hair on your head is insulation against extremes of temperature. Straight hair, with a circular cross-section, is best for this because it traps a layer of air beneath it.

Is it a sign of virility for men to have a hairy chest and body?

No, it bears no relation to sexual desire or performance. It simply depends on how sensitive your hair follicles are to the hormones your body produces, and in most cases this is an inherited characteristic.

"Virility" is a social myth based on the idea that the less you look like a woman (beards, extreme muscular development, etc.) the more sexually aggressive you are and the more women desire you. But it is simply not true. Aggression is usually a sign of inadequacy. Transvestites often have problems with too much body hair, and the shape of your vocal chords has nothing whatever to do with how good you are in bed.

Is it unusual for women to have body hair?

Though some women have very little, many have luxuriant pubic hair with extensive growth on the legs and abdomen and under the armpits. In spite of massive commercial advertising for "beauty aids," shavers and depilatory chemicals, many men still find this an added sexual attraction. After the menopause some women develop facial hair, though it is no more a sign of virility than it is in men.

ERECTIONS

What happens when I get an erection? What makes the penis go hard?

The first stimulus can be purely psychological – sexual thoughts or ideas, or a general mood of feeling "horny" – but it usually involves physical pressure or touch at the same time. Whatever the cause, a special center in the base of the spinal column sends out chemical and nervous signals to the muscles at the base of the penis. Blood vessels open to flood the spongy erectile tissue down either side of it, while other muscles contract to prevent the blood flowing away down the veins. The tissue expands within the sheath of skin, becoming hard, stiffer and usually longer. Other muscles, responding to the increased weight, pull the penis out away from the body at roughly a right angle. The testicles are drawn up toward the abdomen and the scrotum shrinks.

As you get older, the initial stimulus is more likely to be tactile than psychological and the angle of the erection less pronounced.

Can children get erections?

Most males are capable of erection all their lives, from a few days after they are born until well into their eighties and nineties. Adults tend to forget these early experiences because they are not yet associated with sex in our minds, and it often comes as a surprise to parents that very young children naturally have erections. But if they communicate dismay or embarrassment to the child they may condition his attitude to his own body for life.

Is there a female equivalent to erection?

Women also show physical signs of sexual arousal, but these are less obvious and vary considerably from person to person. A woman may become flushed, with heavy breathing or sweating; her clitoris might harden like a miniature penis, though it can be so small as to be almost unnoticeable; her nipples become swollen and erect, especially in the early stages of sexual arousal, though they tend to go down when she becomes more excited; the breasts themselves sometimes swell; and in later stages the outer lips of the vagina open as the inner ones swell up and become darker in color, and the inside lining becomes moist and slippery.

But this is not true of everyone. Some symptoms can be more marked than others and certain women can become sexually excited with few, if any, signs appearing.

The first time I'm with a woman, I have difficulty getting an erection. Is this usual?

There are often minor difficulties at first, but they usually disappear as you get to know one another. In spite of the psychological stimulus, you might be anxious at the back of your mind. Quite apart from embarrassment and possible misunderstandings, you may be worried about contraception, or not being up to it. You are often dealing with the unknown – responses you can't predict, new sensations – and this can only increase your anxiety. It is easy to say "relax," but sometimes very difficult to do. However, it is the only answer, and it is impossible to let yourself go unless (a) you are doing what you *want* rather than what you "ought to," and (b) you take things as they come, instead of worrying about what happens next.

It takes a long time for me to get an erection. Is there a way to speed it up?

Sexual responses vary in their speed, as in most other respects, so maybe you are just one of the "slow movers" who go on longer. Or it may be that you need more physical, rather than psychological, stimulation.

Unless your mental images are roughly matched to your physical sensations, sex can be meaningless. No amount of mechanical manipulation will get you up if your mind is not on it. On the other hand, it's very difficult to get an erection without feedback from your physical senses.

Everyone's body is different and you might be surprised at how little you know about your own responses. The only way to experiment with your own particular combination of chemistry and imagination is through masturbation. It's a good way to find out what turns you on.

I find it difficult to keep an erection. Would artificial aids, such as "cock rings," help to maintain it?

If you find it difficult even when masturbating, then don't force it. If you are all right on your own, but find it difficult with others, the chances are that there is some kind of a psychological blockage which sex aids are unlikely to help. If you only experience problems on some occasions with some people, then those relationships can't be much fun – so why prolong them? If the idea of sex aids turn you on anyway, that's a different matter.

A "cock ring" is a heavy metal ring which slips over the penis when it is flaccid, and then with rather more difficulty over the testicles, until it lies against the body. When the penis is erect the tight ring around its base helps to constrict the blood vessels, and tends to increase and harden the erection. For the same reason, it helps to maintain an erection after an orgasm (in fact it can be more difficult to get off than put on).

Its effectiveness, like any sex aid, depends on your attitude toward it. Some people find them uncomfortable and irritating, while others are aroused by the constant stimulation and the sense of ritual in wearing them.

**I get sexually excited very easily and often find myself with an erection at embarrassing times and places.
Is there a way to prevent this?**

Other people will be much less aware of it than you think, and most of them would consider themselves lucky to be so highly sexed, in spite of occasional embarrassments.

If it is some physical stimulus which causes the problem, you could wear looser clothes or use a desensitizing cream when really necessary. But such hypersensitivity is often the result of frustration. When your sexual drive is not being fulfilled – if, for instance, your only outlet is in unsatisfactory one-night stands – your system nags at you for more and more stimulus as a substitute, until it can almost become an addiction. As this only increases the frustration, it is a vicious circle.

If my penis gets too hard, or I keep an erection for too long, it begins to hurt. Why is this?

The erectile tissue in your penis usually begins to ache if it is kept under pressure for longer than you are used to, with the skin and muscles stretched and the blood vessels swollen. The answer is to take a rest from time to time, change the subject or run it under a cold tap. Once the blood is circulating again the pain vanishes almost immediately, although it may still be tender to the touch.

There is a complaint called *priapism*, usually caused by prostate disease or spinal injury, with which it is impossible to lose an erection. This can be very painful and when the oxygen supply from the blood trapped in the penis is used up the tissue can start to die.

I often wake up in the mornings with an erection. Why is this?

It is possible to go through a full sexual response, including orgasm, while you are asleep. You will usually know if you've had a wet dream, but you may not be aware that you have four or five erections every night. They usually occur during the lighter phases of sleep such as those you experience just before you wake up, so it is not surprising that the morning so often starts with a hard on.

One physical factor which makes it more likely is a full bladder which presses down on your prostate gland and stimulates the sexual organs.

I'm worried that my penis never really gets hard. What can I do about it?

This is another "normal" variation. Many people only get semi-hard erections because the erectile tissue doesn't absorb enough blood or the constricting muscles don't fully hold it back. You can make your penis temporarily stiffer by grasping it firmly around the base or wearing a "cock ring," but there is little point in worrying about it. You are probably not being deprived of any sensations and are just as capable of orgasm.

There is a myth that erection is a measure of excitement. But this is absurd when you remember that early morning erections, without a thought of sex in your head, are often the hardest. If your partner thinks it is lack of response on your part, then show her it is not. She may even prefer an erection which she can partly manipulate.

I understand that an erect penis gets longer, but mine stays the same size and just gets harder. Is there something wrong with it?

No, it simply means that the erectile tissue is not as elastic. It probably also means that your penis is larger than other people's in a relaxed state.

Why does a penis go limp after an orgasm? Is it true that some men can keep an erection even after ejaculation?

When your nerve and hormone systems signal to your body

that the sexual response is over, the muscles relax and the blood drains away from the penis. The erection rapidly reduces to half its size and then, much more slowly, returns to normal. It is easier to hold this stage of semi-erection than regain a full one, and by manual manipulation or leaving the penis in the vagina, it can sometimes be maintained for a long time.

It is largely an involuntary response, but there are certain people who are naturally able (or have taught themselves) to maintain a full erection after they have come, and even achieve something similar to a woman's multiple orgasm. There may well be mind-body exercises, such as yoga, which could teach one the technique, but most of the lucky few admit they have no idea why it happens.

My partner complains about how long it takes me to get another erection after I've ejaculated. What is the usual time?

It can take anything from five minutes to several hours depending on the circumstances. If you are very excited by your partner or change from one partner to another during group sex, it can follow almost immediately. If you are tired or have had a satisfying orgasm, it can take much longer.

SEXUAL ATTRACTION AND INTERCOURSE

What do women find sexually attractive about a man?

The only positive answer is that it is almost certainly not what you think. A recent magazine survey showed that most men have totally the wrong impression of what women find sexually attractive. Top of the women's list of preferences was a small, neat ass, a choice that did's occur on the men's list at all. The men's own idea of their sexual attraction, such as broad shoulders and a handsome face, rated low in the women's preferences.

The truth of the matter is that at a given moment a woman will focus on all sorts of things about you – the line of an eyebrow, an air of assurance, a particular physical type or a look of "little boy" vulnerability. It depends on how she sees you as a stranger, a film star, a fantasy male. It varies with the mood, atmosphere, time and place. It might be the knowledge that you find her sexually attractive, or a sudden mutual leap of recognition, or simply part of a shared companionship.

If you want to be sexually attractive to women, come out about your sexuality, about how you feel about yourself, about the women you want to attract. Let it show in the way you dress, move and express yourself. Be sexy and attractive. And remember that attraction has a passive as well as an active aspect.

Above all, be comfortable. The one sure way to fail is to fake it, because sooner or later you will have to relax. Be yourself and you will soon find how many people are attracted to you.

How important is foreplay in lovemaking?

Foreplay, or what used to be called petting or necking, is any erotic activity short of intercourse. It is more of a social distinction than a biological one because there are no dividing lines except for how far either partner wants to go. The term itself is also misleading because it implies that what comes afterward – intercourse and orgasm – is what really matters. It would be better to call it sex-play or, as some sexologists have suggested, revive the old-fashioned word "pleasuring." This implies a satisfactory activity in its own right, which is what it is. If your sexual activity is goal-oriented and all you are after is an orgasm, you miss out on the real intimacy and meaning (and fun) of sex.

How long should it go on for?

For as long as you enjoy it, or it is practical, or until it becomes unbearable not to go further. It can last for hours, but circumstances usually dictate that you break off or reach a climax in an hour or less. If you are lucky enough to be able to come two or three times there is no need to prolong foreplay, because you can resume it afterward. Ideally you should not only allow time to enjoy yourselves fully, but to rest together afterward.

How will I know when she is ready for intercourse?

She will usually tell you, and if you are enjoying each other it will be obvious. There are the physical signs of arousal, such as increased heart rate and breathing, which show that she has reached the plateau of excitement from which it is possible to have an orgasm. But it is wrong to assume that you have a duty to make decisions of this sort. It is perfectly possible for *her* to take the lead, in which case it is up to you to let her know when *you* are "ready." What usually happens is a mutual surrender to each other, with neither of you aware that a decision has been made.

Is it true that women prefer strong aggressive lovers?

Some women do, and if your partner does she will probably have chosen you for that reason. But she won't expect you suddenly to turn into one if you do not look and act the part. Women are just as likely to prefer a gentle sympathetic person to a confident stud. Women have as wide a variety of tastes as men, and the idea that they all wish to be the passive sex object of virile men is a myth.

But if she has no knowledge of her own sexuality, she may believe it is expected of her. In which case you may find yourselves acting out roles that have nothing to do with what either of you really want.

My partner complains that she is not getting enough. What is the normal frequency of intercourse?

There is a scene in Woody Allen's movie *Annie Hall*, in which he confesses to his psychiatrist what a useless lover he is, barely able to satisfy his girlfriend three or four times a week. At the same time the girlfriend, played by Diane Keaton, is complaining to *her* psychiatrist that she is worn out by the demands of a sex maniac who demands intercourse as often as three or four times a week.

As with most aspects of sex, there are no rules and statistical averages are misleading because they cover such a wide range of behavior. Some people have a more powerful sex drive, or need for reassurance, than others. Passionate lovers may want to satisfy each other several times a day. Long-term relationships, especially those based on ignorance or repetitive patterns, may only need to be expressed sexually once or twice a year. Kinsey's statistics ranged from the man who achieved five orgasms a day for thirty years to the man who had one in all that time.

If your partner complains that she wants it more often, some kind of compromise is the only solution. You might extend your love play so that she can reach an orgasm once or twice before you do, or she might find additional relief by masturbation on her own. If the situation becomes really distressing for either of you, you might reconsider whether you are suited to each other. But try to make sure first that you really know how she feels.

How long should intercourse last?

The easy answer is for as long as it is pleasurable or practical.

Rather like asking how long one should speak to another person, it depends on what your bodies have to say to each other. It can go on for hours or be over in a few minutes. Intercourse is shaped by how much sexual tension you build up and release. The frustrations of a long absence can explode in a brief intense orgasm, while relaxed and experienced partners can extend their sexual play indefinitely. It is not necessary to either partner (let alone both) to reach a climax and much unhappiness has been caused by the belief that this is some sort of "target" to be achieved. It is not. The only reason for sexual intercourse is to enjoy each other and communicate your feelings and emotions to your partner. How you do it, and for how long, is entirely your choice.

Though there is no "normal" form of intercourse, a common pattern of activity might last, say, thirty minutes, with half the time spent in foreplay, kissing, endearments and what used to be called "petting," and the rest at a more intense level of sexual excitement with vaginal and oral intercourse. During this time the man might encourage the woman to two or three orgasms, while holding his own in reserve for the final moments. For instance, he might lie still for a while after entering the vagina when the stimulation is most intense, or slow down when he thinks he is coming. Once he has come, the man usually needs a period of rest to recuperate and this can often be the most tender and intimate moment of all.

Is there a proper time and place for intercourse?

For some people the only place for sex is in bed with one properly licensed member of the opposite sex, at night and with the lights out – but fortunately most of the world would disagree.

In fact there are as many times and places for sexual intercourse as there are for any other human activity, although there is probably a consensus in favor of privacy, enough comfort to relax, enough warmth to take at least some of your clothes off and enough time to enjoy it. The only requirement is that you are sufficiently interested in your partner to become sexually aroused.

Some people prefer it in the dark, out of embarrassment or simply because of the intimacy it brings. Others prefer the pleasure of seeing themselves and looking at each other's bodies. Some like it on the living-room floor in front of a fire, or sharing a bath or shower, or under the sky in open countryside. Some like it behind locked doors; for others there is an added stimulus in an audience, whether or not they take part; and some are turned on by the risk of sexual intercourse in semi-public places. It is surprising where the mood can take you and the opportunity arise.

What is the best position for intercourse?

The geometry of the human body is remarkably flexible and when you are sexually excited almost any part of it can be an "erogenous zone," so there is obviously a wide variety of positions for intercourse. There is no "best" one and each has its own advantages. Most people have their own preference, but if you hold even your ideal position long enough you will end up with cramp. It is much better to keep moving.

You will discover more of the positions from a few minutes free-style wrestling on a bed than from any textbook, but for those who want to check them off against their personal track record, there are several excellent publications illustrating sexual positions. And, of course, there is the *Kama Sutra*, which includes additional categories for the various sizes of organs and apertures, marital status and your poetic frame of mind at the time. Then you might add the possible positions for all the variations of oral, anal and intercrural intercourse and mutual masturbation. . . . Well, by that time who's counting?

Treating it as a numbers game can be silly, but there are definite advantages to experimenting. Some of the "standard" positions are positively uncomfortable and make it difficult to control one's movements – or move at all.

Once again, there are no rules, but there are one or two points worth bearing in mind.

Many people find it difficult to reach an orgasm unless they are in control of their own body movements, and positions in which both partners are free to make rhythmic hip movements allow for more flexible responses.

It is preferable that one partner does not have to bear the full weight of the other's body for too long. If you are on top, you must usually prop yourself up with your arms, which means that you cannot use your hands to caress or stimulate your partner.

Many people find it desirable to see their partner's body during intercourse, so don't be too quick to turn the light out.

During prolonged intercourse almost any position can become tiring. You may be feeling fine, but it is not much use if her attention is entirely devoted to excruciating pins and needles.

Although it is often more comfortable to lie down, it is by no means necessary. There are many ways of having sex sitting down, standing or partly reclining.

There is greater depth of penetration if the woman bends her legs at an angle to her body, or if the partners' bodies are at an angle to each other, like a cross. Rear entry also allows great depth of penetration provided that neither partner is overweight.

I've heard that the "missionary" position is the proper one for sexual intercourse. What is it and why is it called that?

The "missionary" position is where the man lies full length on top of the woman with his penis inserted from the front. The name probably derives from the fact that it is the sort of position which a prudish or inhibited couple might adopt, with the woman's "passive" role firmly established and the man doing all the work. At the same time there is not much scope for sinful pleasure, because either the man's body is crushing his partner or his arms are occupied in bearing his weight.

Apart from this it is a reasonably comfortable position which allows the man adequate penetration and provides indirect stimulation to the region of the woman's clitoris by pressure of the pubic bones, though it can be improved if the woman raises her knees and spreads her legs so that the man can lie between them.

My partner prefers to be on top. Does this mean that she is dominating and that I am weak?

No, it probably just means that she prefers that position. It can be a very satisfying one for a woman, where she can control the stimulation of her vaginal area and finds it easy to bring herself to an orgasm. It is also very pleasant for the man, especially if he wishes to conserve his energies for a later orgasm. He is relaxed, with both hands free, and if she is sitting astride him, he has her whole body to play with and can even stimulate her clitoris with his hands during intercourse.

There is no social status in sex, where "surrender" can be the most positive act and "breaking the rules" an intimate conspiracy. So "weakness" and "strength" have no meaning in the usual sense. One of the main pleasures in sex is to give pleasure, and to share in your partner's excitement. But if domination fantasies play a part in your relationship, they can easily be adapted to circumstances by assuming (a) that you have given her permission to enjoy herself, or (b) that she has ordered you to do it.

If you still don't enjoy it, then don't do it.

Is the rear-entry position abnormal?

Questions about what is "normal" are usually hedged about with so many qualifications that they become meaningless. But for once it is possible to give a positive answer, because one of the most unusual things about human sexual intercourse is that we *don't* use the rear-entry position. Most of the animal kingdom does and we are the only mammals, apart from whales, dolphins and (very occasionally) monkeys, who have face-to-face sexual intercourse.

Whether sitting, bending, lying side-by-side or on all fours, there is a wide variety of positions in which the penis can enter the vagina from behind, and they are all worth trying. The rear-entry position not only provides effective penetration, but is extremely satisfying for both men and women. It leaves the hands free for other stimulation and, by slightly twisting the bodies (as if she were sitting across your lap, so to speak) it is still possible to have face-to-face contact.

Is depth of penetration important?

Depth of penetration is important to the man, but less to the woman. Her sensitive areas are around the opening of the vagina, not deep inside, so that the angle of entry, the degree of movement from side to side and stimulation of the clitoris are more important to her satisfaction. It is not even necessary for the penis to be the only means of stimulation. Surveys have shown that most women achieve their most intense orgasms by manual masturbation and there are many ways in which your hands can be busy in the same area.

But partial penetration can be very frustrating for the man and a bit of experimenting can usually satisfy the needs of both partners.

Do women like you to thrust gently or hard?

It depends on the mood you are both in. There is a time for gentle playfulness, just as there are times to surrender to your instincts. It is usually better to start slowly and build to a climax, but there are many intermediate stages at which you can ease up or stop and start again. The most important factor is the smoothness and rhythm of your movements, and the ability to synchronize them to those of your partner. Unintentional rough handling or clumsiness can make sexual arousal difficult and intercourse actually painful, so if in doubt, be gentle. Holding back a little can even intensify the experience.

I've heard of yoga intercourse which can go on for hours. Is there any truth in this?

Yes, it is perfectly true. Eastern cultures have taken a more civilized attitude toward sex than our own and long ago integrated it as an art form in their society and religion. One result is that they have learned to combine imagination and physical sensations in a single experience. If you really understand and control your body the slightest touch can be an intense experience. Just try touching the tips of someone's fingers as slowly and lightly as possible, or gently stroking the fine hairs on a sensitive place without touching the skin, and you will discover how feelings can be amplified to almost unendurable pleasure by the mind. With practice it is possible to achieve a full orgasm without physical or visual stimulation of any kind and some experienced yogi have learned to control their internal muscles to such an extent that they can actually draw water up their penises into their bladders.

One form of yoga involves sexual intercourse virtually without movement. The woman sits astride the man with his penis in her vagina and both partners go into a form of sexual trance or meditation which can last for hours and be intensely satisfying without either of them having an orgasm. But it takes practice, so don't be disappointed by poor results at first if you decide to try it.

Is it important to come together, at the same moment?

There is no particular significance in a simultaneous orgasm, unless it has some special meaning for both partners. Many people prefer to reach their climax in sequence so that each can enjoy the other's orgasm to the full.

There is also a practical reason for taking it in turn, because men and women require a different kind of stimulation at the critical moment. Men often like to stop moving when the flood gates open inside them and they feel the muscles pumping out the ejaculation. Women, on the other hand, do not experience this internal hydraulic pressure and usually prefer the stimulation to continue during their orgasm. Some couples place great importance on the woman having an orgasm before the man because, if he comes first, he may feel too tired and his penis be too limp to continue, leaving the woman unsatisfied.

But there is no overriding *need* to synchronize orgasms. In fact, rules and standards of "success" like this are usually a sign of insecurity. There's always next time.

ORGASM

I know what it feels like, but what actually happens during an orgasm?

The feelings are what really matter. However, this is the sequence of physical events, which occur in several distinct phases.

When the body systems become sexually excited, by a mental or physical stimulus, the heartbeat increases to twice the normal rate and the muscles of the lower abdomen become tense. The sphincter muscles of the anus and bladder tighten, the scrotum shrinks and the testicles are raised up to the body. The blood vessels from the penis are constricted so that they act like a one-way valve, allowing blood in but not out. The spongy material in the penis is inflated and, as the blood pressure increases, becomes stiff and hard. The contracted muscles hold the penis out at an angle to the body.

At a certain point the heart rate levels off (at about 120 beats a minute) and this excited "plateau" stage can be maintained for long periods, or lost and regained many times, without an orgasm. If the excitement increases, other changes occur. The testicles swell up and are drawn still closer to the body. The diameter of the penis increases and the tip sometimes enlarges and changes to a darker color. Finally, when a critical threshold of pressures, rhythms and hormones is reached, an orgasm is triggered off.

As an orgasm approaches, the heartbeat increases again, up to $2\frac{1}{2}$ times the normal rate; breathing becomes heavy; and there can be a flushing of the skin, especially around the neck and forehead, and sweating all over the body. The sperm and other seminal fluids build up pressure in the valves around the top of the urethra. The whole body reaches a pitch of hypersensitivity and activity, with involuntary convulsive movements and sounds such as sighs and groans.

With all systems go, the final signal sets off an automatic series of muscular contractions around the urethra; the prostate, like a finely tuned carburetor, injects the right mixture of seminal fluids down the penis. There are usually three or four bursts of semen at intervals of 0.8 seconds, ejaculated with some force from a few inches to several feet. These are usually followed by weaker and less regular contractions.

The final "resolution" stage is a gradual winding down. The sex flushes disappear and as the blood pressure and heart rate drop, the penis rapidly deflates to about $1\frac{1}{2}$ times its usual size. From then on it slowly reduces to normal.

There are wide differences between people's sexual responses, and not everyone will experience all the phenomena. Each stage can be prolonged under the right circumstances. Equally, it is possible to ejaculate – in a mechanical way – without even having an erection.

What does sperm consist of, and how much is produced in an orgasm?

The amount of semen ejaculated during an orgasm varies between 2.2 and 6.5 milliliters, but on average it is about 3.5 milliliters – a small coffeespoonful.

It is usually a milky opalescent fluid with a distinct smell (from the prostate fluid) and a bitter-sweet taste that varies between individuals. The liquid consists of different elements, which are discharged in a carefully timed sequence.

First there is a preliminary clear fluid which trickles from the Cowper's gland into the urethra and neutralizes any acidity left there by urine. This fluid sometimes emerges as drops on the tip of the penis before orgasm. Secondly, the prostate releases a wave of thin milky fluid, which makes up about 40 percent of the ejaculation and is the medium in which the sperm will swim. Then come the sperm themselves – between 150 and 400 million of them, though they only represent about 2 percent of the seminal fluid. Finally, the seminal vesicles beside the prostate emit a flood of sticky yellow fluid, which is mostly milk-sugar and which acts as a food supply for the sperm on their journey.

Although most of these fluids are released separately, it is important to realize that there are fertile sperm in all of them. Last-minute withdrawal of the penis is a risky form of contraception since it is quite possible for a woman to conceive from a tiny drop of Cowper's fluid before (or even without) a full orgasm.

Does an orgasm feel the same for a woman?

The nature of the female orgasm has been argued about for many years by doctors and psychologists. It was once thought that women did not have orgasms at all, in spite of very obvious evidence to the contrary. Then it was assumed that the orgasm was focused on the clitoris, like a scaled-down version of a man's. Later on the pioneer sexual studies of the 1950s and 1960s showed conclusively that the female orgasm involved muscular contractions and other symptoms deep in the vagina. This started a debate about the relative merits of "clitoral" and "vaginal" orgasms – an argument which was bound to be inconclusive, because they are, in effect, the same thing.

In fact, the biological changes during female orgasms are much the same as in men, though the foreplay, erogenous zones and mental images may feel quite different. The same stages occur, although women generally take longer to reach a "plateau" and can maintain it at a higher level for longer. They are also more inclined to show symptoms such as a flushed appearance, sweating and heavy breathing. The increase in the heart rate is the same and even the waves of muscular contractions through the vagina are synchronized to the same intervals as those of the man.

What differences there are seem to be subjective ones. The male orgasm tends to be more rhythmic and muscular, with an intense feeling of the build-up and release of fluids, centered on the genitals. Not having the same hydraulics, women do not experience the same physical release of an ejaculation. Their orgasm is a single experience involving two possible sets of muscular contractions, one around the vagina and the other deep in the chest. When they happen together the two sensations are linked in an explosive feeling through the whole body, but usually one or the other occurs on its own.

It is possible for men to experience an orgasm through their whole body, but the technique requires a certain self-control. The trick is to totally relax one's body (every muscle of it) once an orgasm is inevitable, but before you actually ejaculate. It takes considerable willpower at such a tense moment, but the feeling is worth it.

What are different forms of female orgasm?

The most common is the *vulval orgasm*, first studied by Masters and Johnson. This involves involuntary rhythmic contractions of muscles in the walls of the vulva, starting in the outer third of the vagina and spreading upward to the uterus, and sometimes accompanied by muscular contractions in the buttocks and legs. Although this form of orgasm can be produced by vaginal intercourse, it is not dependant on penetration and can easily be produced by other methods including masturbation and clitoral stimulation.

The second is the *uterine orgasm*, which usually results from very deep penetration when the penis jostles the wall of the cervix at the back of the vagina. The feeling is transmitted up through the abdomen to the muscles of the diaphragm and throat. These eventually go into an involuntary spasm, with the holding of a deep breath followed by a violent exhalation of air and an orgasm.

These are only two aspects of the female orgasm and there may be other forms, in both men and women. In theory, any set of involuntary muscles can be stimulated into a temporary spasm, and the feedback to the brain which creates the "feeling" is far from clear. Since the diaphragm and throat muscles are common to both sexes, it may even be possible for men to experience an equivalent to the uterine orgasm.

I've heard that women can have multiple orgasm. Is this true? Can men do it?

Unlike men, women have the ability to maintain their sexual "plateau" after they have come, so they can experience several orgasms in succession. They can usually achieve three to five in a few minutes, although as many as twelve in an hour have been recorded.

Although it is rare, it has been known for some men (by practice, yoga or good luck) to be able to do the same and achieve several orgasms without losing their erection. But it *is* rare, and no one expects it of you.

Can men really come four or five times in as many hours? What is the average performance?

The British therapist, Robert Chartham, who claims to have multiple orgasms himself, has recorded one twenty-two-year-old male who achieved eight orgasms in $2\frac{1}{2}$ hours, and an astonishing twenty-three-year-old who managed ten separate orgasms in eighty minutes without losing his erection.

But don't be discouraged. In a couple of hours most of us can manage one orgasm, some a second and a few of us can make it three or four times. However, intercourse is not a competition, and frequency is not a vital statistic. A single intense orgasm can be fully satisfying.

I'm worried about coming too fast. Is there anything I can do about it?

By far the most common cause of premature ejaculation is fear of premature ejaculation – the anxiety that arises from placing too much importance on satisfying your partner's needs. If you get worried about coming too soon, you probably will.

There are mildly anesthetic creams available which can be applied to the penis to make it less sensitive. But it is better to treat it as a game rather than a problem. Hold back on the foreplay and concentrate on your partner. Stop and take a rest if you feel your orgasm is imminent: it's not necessary (or necessarily better) to make love continuously. Talk or joke about it instead of apologizing.

Premature ejaculation can also be caused by prolonged abstinence or simply by inexperience (it takes time to learn how to pace yourself). Or it may be a matter of habit, reflecting the urgency of semi-private meeting places or the need for speed with prostitutes.

How can I tell if a woman is faking an orgasm?

By getting to know her.

In the right circumstances it is comparatively easy for either sex to fake it. But if she *is* simulating, it is probably because you both place too much importance on the orgasm. Does she think it is required as "proof" of something? Or do you? Relaxed sexual play, without trying to reach climax, can be one of the closest ways for human beings to interrelate.

Can she feel my ejaculation?

Outside her body, yes. Inside, during vaginal intercourse, it's unlikely unless she is very sensitive or you have a formidable ejaculation. But body language is very expressive, and with so many feelings and sensations pouring in, she probably knows exactly when you are coming.

Sometimes she has these orgasms which shake her so much she becomes hysterical, and it frightens me. Is this usual?

Orgasm is a powerful experience, and may be powerfully expressed. It is nothing to be frightened of. Some women remain almost silent during orgasm, others express their pleasure noisily, with laughter, cries or even tears. It is probably a matter of upbringing as much as anything else. Let yourself go and express *your* feelings too. Ride it together and enjoy it. Your response can enhance or destroy her excitement and pleasure.

My partner never achieves orgasm. Is this usual? What can I do about it? Does it affect her physically?

Virtually all women are capable of it, but many are inhibited by prejudices acquired as children or by simple ignorance about their own bodies.

What this question usually means, however, is "my partner never reaches orgasm during intercourse *with me*" – which is a very different matter. It is also a very common one. One of the most distressing of all sexual statistics is that between 11 percent and 25 percent of married women (depending on the age group) never experience an orgasm during marital intercourse.

Communication is nearly always at the root of the problem. Have you bothered to find out what really turns her on? You could experiment with and extend your foreplay – which is half the fun of sex anyway. Maybe you are not giving her, time to work up to it. Maybe you have got her too worried to relax into it. Maybe you should try new positions.

Although the clitoris is the most sensitive female sex organ, some forms of intercourse – including the "missionary" position – do not directly stimulate it. Encourage her to let you masturbate her, and when you do something she likes the feeling of, get her to let you know.

Failure to reach orgasm will have no direct physical effects, but if it causes either of you frustration or anxiety it can be as damaging, physically and psychologically, as any form of stress.

My testicles feel tight after orgasm. Why is this?

One sign of sexual arousal is that the testicles are raised and the scrotum retracts. If they have been like this for some time, they tend to feel tight: but a little gentle massage after orgasm will usually relax them. A similar "blocked-up" feeling can occur when you have been very worked up but do not have an orgasm, and the glands feel as if they are bursting with unreleased sperm. The solution in this case is obvious.

Should I leave her alone after an orgasm, or go on making love gently?

It is more likely that she will be the one who wants to go on making love, because women are much slower to come down from the plateau of sexual excitement than men, and the man will often collapse in satisfied exhaustion leaving his partner still partially aroused. So it is usually something of a compromise. For instance, if the orgasm occurs during vaginal intercourse, there is no need for the man to withdraw immediately and his partner can continue to manipulate herself.

Certain parts of the body, especially the penis, can feel extremely sensitive and tender after an orgasm, but gently caressing or kissing or simply holding each other makes the pleasure last that much longer.

After sex I feel drained and depressed. Is this usual?

The period after an orgasm is sometimes accompanied by what doctors call *post-coitum triste*. It usually comes about because the everyday concerns, or guilt about the sex itself, come rushing back into your mind and your natural exhaustion and vulnerability heighten the feelings of anxiety or depression.

But it depends entirely on the circumstances and your frame of mind. If you are relaxed and secure, you feel pleasantly exhausted ʾather than "drained" and instead of anxiety you can experience a shared tenderness and intimacy as satisfying as any orgasm.

Contraception and Conception

It is possible to divide sexual activity into biological reproduction on the one hand, and all other aspects of intercourse, including love, on the other. "Metasex" is a term recently coined to describe the huge realms of erotic behaviour not directly concerned with reproduction. Metasex is for pleasure, for expressing affection, for exchanging energy and for communication.

However, in this section we cover reproductive sex, starting with menstruation and including the processes involved in conception, ways of helping nature and methods of preventing the biological chain reaction taking place.

MENSTRUATION

Why do women menstruate, and what happens?

Menstruation is part of the regular cycle which occurs in a woman's body from the age of about twelve to forty-seven.

The sequence begins in the woman's ovaries. These contain about 350,000 immature eggs, but only about 375 of them mature, one at a time, at monthly intervals during her life. Each mature egg is released down the Fallopian tube, which runs from its particular ovary to the uterus or womb. The chemical hormones which trigger the release of the egg also signal to the uterus to prepare for its arrival, which it does by growing a thick lining of cells. If the egg happens to be fertilized on its journey down the tube, it will stick to this lining in the uterus which then becomes the placenta through which the fetus is fed by the mother. But if the egg is not fertilized, it simply passes through the uterus and disappears in the normal vaginal discharge. In this case, the hormones cease to manufacture the lining and it is discarded in turn. The discharge of these fragments of cell lining, amounting to between two and four tablespoons of fluid, and the feelings produced by the hormone changes, are known as menstruation. Once the system is cleared out, the cycle starts again.

What are sanitary napkins and tampons?

During menstruation most women take steps to prevent the accidental staining of clothes or bedsheets with blood, by inserting a small absorbent tube (a tampon) into their vagina, or by wearing an absorbent pad (a sanitary napkin) over it.

How often does it occur, and how regular is it?

The whole cycle, including ovulation and menstruation, is regulated by hormones to roughly twenty-eight days, though some women have cycles as short as nineteen days or as long as thirty-seven days. If a woman lives a steady and contented life, her periods can tick away as regularly as clockwork, but they can easily be disturbed. Emotional stress can alter the pattern and it is even possible for her to miss a period and then resume them later. Menstruation stops during pregnancy and often takes some time to start again after the baby is born. It finally ceases altogether when the woman reaches her menopause.

What is the menopause?

At some point in her life between the late thirties and fifties (but usually about the age of forty-seven), a woman's hormones "turn off." There is no further menstruation, the ovulation cycle stops and she can no longer have children.

It is the way which nature has evolved to ensure that children have parents who are young and healthy enough to look after them and that they don't inherit damaged genetic material. But although it is a natural process, it can bring radical and distressing changes to a woman's life. The upset balance of her body chemistry produces emotional moods and she may feel depressed that she is no longer a "real" woman. But it does not affect her sexual needs and pleasures and she is still a complete person in every other respect.

Are there regular cycles in a man's sexuality?

There is very little recorded evidence of regular cycles. Men's sexual activity and biological systems, including the production of sperm and the capacity for orgasm, are more or less continuous. But most doctors concede that very little is known about the wider influences on sexual rhythms. The lunar cycle has a marked effect on women's sexuality and there may well be a similar but milder influence on men which shows itself in increased hormone production and heightened sexual awareness. In addition to this, if you share a close relationship with a woman, it is difficult not to respond to the rhythms of her life.

Your sexual feelings may even be influenced by long-term seasonal changes, according to some recent research. Analysis of birth statistics in France has shown, for instance, that it is not the spring when "a young man's fancy turns to love," but the fall, because a larger number of children were born in the summer months.

The question of the male "menopause" is dealt with later, but it seems to be more a matter of social and psychological pressures than physical change. In sexual matters, though, it is always difficult to tell where psychology ends and biology begins.

Is it true that menstruation makes women depressed and irritable? If so, why?

The hormones which trigger off menstruation tend to have side effects on other body systems. For two or three days beforehand, it is common for a woman to suffer from back ache, headaches and mild bouts of depression. She has probably learned to cope with this in such a way that it passes almost unnoticed, but she still has the right to expect some tolerance and sympathy. Emotional tension and anxiety in her everyday life will certainly exaggerate the symptoms.

Sometimes the chemical imbalance is so marked that the woman suffers a complete personality change. This syndrome, known as "premenstrual depression," has only recently been pinpointed and analyzed, but it is obvious that many women suffer from it. The effects last for up to two weeks. The physical aches and pains, including lumpiness in the breast tissues, which can become very sore and tender, are all more extreme and are accompanied by psychological symptoms. The woman can become moody and irritable, sensitive to the most casual remark, quick to anger and very depressed. It does not happen every period, but when it does it can cause considerable distress to the woman and her family.

In the past, women with premenstrual tension have been treated with tranquilizers and advice to pull themselves together, but there are now special therapy clinics in most major cities which offer more practical help to women who suffer from it.

Is it possible to have intercourse during a woman's periods?

It is certainly possible, and many women are more sexually sensitive at this time. It is also one of the few times when intercourse is perfectly safe without any form of contraception. Whether or not you are put off it for aesthetic reasons is another matter. Intercourse will usually be accompanied by the presence of blood, and many people are upset by the mere sight of this. But in other respects it feels the same for both of you.

My partner thinks she is pregnant because her period is two weeks late. Is she right?

A missed period is certainly the first sign of a pregnancy, so she may be right. But it doesn't always mean this. The regular cycle of periods can be upset for a variety of reasons and there is no way either of you can tell without medical tests such as a urine analysis. Excitement or anxiety, or a change of lifestyle such as travel, can all delay periods or bring them on early. The biological clocks which run our systems are more flexible than mechanical ones. It has even been found that women who live together tend to subconsciously adjust their periods until they are synchronized with each other.

But if you think she might be pregnant, there is no point in hoping or worrying or trusting to luck. It is easy to have it checked out by a pregnancy service or clinic.

Can the Pill or other contraceptives affect a woman's menstruation?

The Pill has a marked effect on menstruation and the rest of the sexual cycle. It can be used to regulate it or suppress it altogether, and the way this works is explained later. Other forms of contraception have little or no effect.

CONTRACEPTION

Is contraception the man's or the woman's responsibility?

In any sexual relationship, no matter how brief, it is essential for both of you to know what safeguards the other is taking. Even if you have had a sterilization operation (*vasectomy*) and are certain in your own mind that there is no risk of pregnancy, your partner may still be anxious and worried unless she knows. If she doesn't mention it, you must.

In practical terms the "responsibility" varies from one relationship to another. If, for instance, the woman is already on the Pill, there is no need for the man to do anything further. But with less reliable contraception, some people prefer more than one method. If the couple are relying on the withdrawal technique, for example, or the man is wearing a condom, then the woman may wish to take the additional precaution of using a spermicidal foam.

If you enjoy a busy sex life with a number of partners it is very inconsiderate not to use contraception yourself on a regular basis.

Does it lessen sexual pleasure?

In the case of the Pill, IUD and vasectomy there is absolutely no physical sensation, so you can forget about the subject and enjoy yourselves. Even in the case of the more cumbersome methods contraception needn't lessen your pleasure or excitement provided it is incorporated into your love play. If you have to break off to go to the bathroom to fit a condom it can destroy the whole mood, whereas it can actually increase the pleasure to make a game of it and let your partner fit it for you. In the same way foams and jellies, like lubricants, can be fun in themselves.

The one thing that interferes with sexual pleasure more than anything else, is feeling guilty that one hasn't taken precautions and worrying whether the other has done so.

What are the methods and how safe are they?

There are roughly ten methods of contraception, which can be arranged in three groups in ascending order of reliability. The first group has a safety record of only 70 percent to 80 percent effectiveness – the douche (with only a one-in-three chance of preventing a pregnancy), the rhythm method, the use of spermicidal jelly and withdrawal (or *coitus interruptus*).

The next group is roughly 85 percent to 90 percent effective. It includes the sheath or condom, the diaphragm (or "Dutch cap") and spermicidal foam.

The last group has a safety record which gives you less than a 5 percent chance of a pregnancy. These "safe" methods include IUD (inter-uterine devices), the Pill, and safest of all, sterilization.

Is there an "ideal" form of contraception?

An ideal method would put the onus of responsibility on those who actually *wanted* to conceive, in the form of an easily applied (and preferably self-induced), cheap, fully reversible (but otherwise secure) sterilization which interferes as little as possible with the natural metabolism and produces no other side effects.

Male vasectomy comes closest to this definition, but it requires a medical operation to apply and is not always reversible. Current medical research is concentrating on the first two requirements by developing the male hormone-based pill and improving the female version.

What is the douche method?

The douche method relies on washing out the vagina immediately after intercourse, preferably using a douche bag or bidet. It needs enough self-control for instant action and is very unreliable because of the difficulty in ensuring that all the sperm are removed – but it is better than nothing.

We use the rhythm method, but I think my partner's got it wrong. How does it work?

The *rhythm method* relies on the fact that there is only a short period in a woman's sexual cycle when there is a mature egg in her body available for fertilization. This is during the twenty-four hours or so, after each monthly ovulation, while the egg is passing down the Fallopian tube to the uterus. Ovulation usually takes place on the fifteenth day of the twenty-eight-day cycle, but it can vary over a period of five days so these must also be considered "unsafe." Since sperm can survive for up to seventy-two hours in her body, and slow-moving eggs can be fertilized up to twenty-four hours later than expected, another five days has to be added to the period when conception can occur. Outside this period you are safe. In theory at any rate, sexual intercourse cannot cause a pregnancy for the nine days after the start of one menstruation and nine days before the next. But sexual cycles vary enormously and it is easy to be caught out.

There is one way of checking each cycle which makes the method more reliable, called the *temperature-rhythm method*. A woman shows a sudden rise in body temperature during the day of ovulation which is caused by a sudden rise in production of the hormone progesterone. By the time this temperature is recorded, the fertile period is usually over and it signals the start of the "safe" period. But there is still no way of knowing for certain how long after menstruation the next ovulation might occur. The effectiveness of the method depends on the woman keeping very careful records of her periods and temperatures, and being sure that they are predictable. It also depends on your being able to control yourself at the same monthly intervals, so this form of statistical contraception can be both unreliable and frustrating.

Is "coitus interruptus" safe? Is it possible for a fertile amount of semen to leak out before an orgasm occurs?

Withdrawal can be an even more frustrating form of contraception than the rhythm method, although it is marginally more effective, with an 18 percent as opposed to a 24 percent chance of conception.

The drawback is in applying the method at all. If you prefer to achieve orgasm by vaginal intercourse it can require a superhuman effort of will to pull out in time, and the safety figures only apply to those who make it. The method is easier to apply if your lovemaking does not rely on vaginal orgasm, and you are satisfied with other forms of intercourse.

However determined and single-minded you are, the method is inherently unreliable because sperm can be passed through the penis before you finally ejaculate. The longer your sexual activity and the closer you come to orgasm, the more likely it is for the odd hundred thousand sperm to bridge the gap. It is possible for a drop of seminal fluid to leak out before you come – or even have a full erection.

How effective are spermicidal foams and creams?

Considerable research has gone into producing chemicals which destroy sperm on contact, and in ideal conditions they work well. What makes them relatively ineffective as a means of contraception is the difficulty of ensuring that necessary contact. Even if the internal surfaces of the vagina are covered with it, there is no guarantee that the sperm will not just swim past. For this reason the aerosol foams which fill the vaginal cavity and block the entrance to the uterus are the best, if the most messy.

The other forms are the suppositories and tablets, which are supposed to dissolve in the vagina but are not very reliable; and the creams and jellies. These are most effective used in conjunction with sheaths and diaphragms, particularly if you put some in the end of the condom before you roll it on.

As with all chemicals used for contraception, or as sex aids, there is a danger of allergies. So it is wise to check with your doctor first, or at least to experiment a little, before smearing them all over yourself.

I have heard of women having a coil fitted. What is it and how does it work?

The *inter-uterine device,* or IUD, or coil, is a form of non-chemical contraception consisting of a piece of metal, like wire, twisted into a variety of shapes such as loops and spirals, and inserted into the woman's uterus through the opening in the cervix. It works by preventing a fertilized egg from attaching itself to the lining and growing into a fetus. Instead it behaves like an unfertilized one, passes straight through and is discharged from the vagina in the normal way.

The IUD is very effective, with less than a 5 percent chance of conception. It interferes with none of the other body functions, periods occur as usual and most women prefer it to any other form of contraception. Should she wish to conceive at any time, the coil is as easy to remove as it is to insert. However, it does have some drawbacks. Some women do not like the idea of having an instrument permanently inside them; others find it acutely uncomfortable or cannot keep it in place; and since individuals require different shapes it often takes several "fittings" to select the most suitable design. In the case of an accidental pregnancy they can cause miscarriages. But when they are suitable and fit properly, contraception requires no effort of memory or willpower and the woman can forget she is even wearing it.

What is the Pill? Is it as reliable and safe as they say?

The oral hormone-based contraceptive for women – the famous "Pill" – was hailed as the solution to all contraceptive problems when it was introduced in the fifties. It was the first openly available, cheap, reliable form of birth control and rapidly became the major form of contraception. It is no exaggeration to say that it brought about a social revolution in many Western countries and gave millions of women the freedom to explore their own sexuality for the first time. But so much evidence has accumulated in the last few years of its long-term dangers and unpleasant side effects that early opinions about it are being drastically revised.

The pills, containing synthetic versions of two female hormones, estrogen and progesterone, are sold in carefully numbered packs which last a month and the woman takes one a day. The chemicals are produced naturally in the woman's body at regular intervals to trigger off the sexual cycle and the sequence of other hormones which carry it through. They are also produced continuously during pregnancy to block the sequence and prevent ovulation and menstruation occurring. The Pill simulates these "pregnancy" conditions, so that no eggs are available to be fertilized. There is no need to keep taking the pill during the safe period, so the packs either run out or contain dummy pills for one week in the month so the woman can have her period. If the pill is taken continuously there is no menstruation, but this completely blocks her natural rhythms and can cause distressing psychological symptoms in addition to other harmful side effects.

The pills come in three forms: the *combination pill,* which contains a substantial amount of both hormones; the *sequential pill,* which mimics the natural cycle better, with estrogen in most of the tablets and progesterone only added to a few; and the *mini-pill,* which has a lower dosage of hormones altogether and no estrogen. The combination pill is the most effective but produces the worst side effects, and the mini-pill causes the least damage.

The effects on individual metabolisms vary, but when a woman first goes on the pill she can suffer from headaches, sore and swollen breasts, nausea, vaginal bleeding and fatness due to the body retaining more water. These symptoms can be accompanied by mood alterations and a reduction of sexual desire. While these effects tend to disappear after the first three months, many women accept them as the more or less permanent price of peace of mind.

Are there any long-term effects?

It is now recognized that the continuous intake of hormones which the body doesn't need can have very serious long-term effects. The most likely of these is heart trouble. Both estrogen and progesterone can cause blood clotting and an increase in blood pressure after five years' use. In women with certain blood groups they can produce thrombosis, and the overall figures are ominous. Recent statistics show that any woman who has ever taken the Pill *at any time* is five times more likely to die of coronary disease than a non-Pill-user. If she has been on the Pill for more than five years the death rate increases to ten times that of non-users. (Royal College of General Practioners report, *Lancet*, Oct. 8. 1977.)

The risk to women over forty is now considered unacceptable, and even those over thirty-five, who combine some other risk factor such as smoking, are being advised to stop using the Pill.

In fairness one should add that millions of women find no difficulty in using it and many people would argue that its advantages vastly outweigh the risks. Research is being carried out on improved forms of hormone-based contraception and the reduced-dosage pills will probably reduce the risk, but it is obviously important that women should obtain medical advice before using it and receive regular medical check-ups while they are on it.

What is sterilization?

Sterilization involves surgically cutting some of the tubing which links the sex organs and, either by removing a section or tying off the ends, preventing the system from operating. The operation in men (*vasectomy*) prevents the sperm from reaching the penis and in women it blocks the passage of the mature egg down the Fallopian tube. For women this means a few days in the hospital and an operation under general anesthetic, but for men it is a much simpler process taking only a few minutes and a local anesthetic.

It should by rights be called infertilization rather than sterilization, because the aim of doctors now is to develop a reversible operation. If the man should want it, new surgical techniques mean that vasectomy stands a reasonable chance of being reversed, although the equivalent female operation is less likely to be successful.

Sterilization is the most secure form of contraception and there is an increasing demand for it among middle-aged couples or parents who do not want any more children. But the need for surgery and its apparent permananence still put many people off.

What about vasectomy? Will it make me a eunuch?

Vasectomy is designed for one purpose – to ensure that your semen contains no sperm. It is not castration, nothing is removed, your voice stays in the same register and you are still capable of what feels like a full orgasm.

The operation involves a small incision in the scrotum so that the doctor can reach the vas deferens tube which carries the sperm from the testes up to the urethra. This is cut and the ends sealed with small clamps (if the operation is to be reversible). The whole thing is painless and heals without even a scar to boast about.

It must be recognized by anyone agreeing to a vasectomy that it *may* prove irreversible. In the present state of medical knowledge that is the price of 100 percent safe contraception.

Are there any new forms of contraception being developed?

One of the most promising new developments is a device which takes all the guess-work out of the rhythm method. Instead of having to work out an elaborate formula from a calendar, it enables a woman to know *exactly* when she is ovulating and therefore to pinpoint the two or three days each month when she is likely to conceive. The device, which will eventually be available as an instrument about the size of a pocket calculator, analyzes the consistency of cervical mucus, which becomes more fluid at the peak periods of fertility. The *mucothermic method,* as it's called, combines these measurements with a daily temperature record to provide a remarkably safe and accurate form of natural contraception.

Strange as it seems, another new development may one day make it possible for a woman to be vaccinated against pregnancy. Vaccines are normally used to alert the body's defenses to attack and destroy intruders such as disease bacteria, but the contraceptive vaccine involves the risky step of producing antibodies to attack one of the body's own natural hormones. The hormone, human chorionic gonadotrophin (HCG), is produced by the egg itself once it is implanted and plays a critical role in allowing it to remain fixed to the wall of the uterus. If it is eliminated by antibodies, the egg is discharged as if it were infertile, along with the uterine lining, in the usual way. Unfortunately HCG is almost indistinguishable from the main female sex hormone progesterone, and very little is known of its other possible functions, so the vaccine could produce serious and unforeseen side-effects.

Many years of research in America, Australia, India and the UK, have gone into producing a selective antibody which can tell HCG from progesterone. In 1975, some successful animal experiments were carried out in America and the following year the Indian government sponsored trials of the new vaccine on both sterilized and fertile women. These proved unsuccessful and have since been criticized as being premature. Other animal experiments, with monkeys, have shown that the vaccine works provided that there are frequent "booster" shots, but that there are difficulties in reversing the process to make the animals fertile again. However, scientists remain optimistic, research continues, and it seems likely that clinical trials of the contraceptive vaccine will soon begin in earnest.

I've heard they are developing a male pill. What is the current status of it?

The design of an oral contraceptive for men has proved far more difficult than the women's Pill. Unlike the female sexual cycle, the male system does not have a sequence of events which can be interrupted at a single point. It's a continuous process, which requires a permanent chemical imbalance to suppress. The problem has been to find a precise enough hormone dosage, like a selective weed killer, to render the sperm infertile without producing drastic side effects on the metabolism.

The results of current research are ambiguous, and it seems unlikely that a male pill will be available in the immediate future.

I sometimes get carried away and forget to think about contraception. Is there an effective way of preventing conception after intercourse has taken place?

There is no guaranteed way of retrieving the situation, but you can always hope. If it has gone that far, and it is that serious, the best thing to do is for your partner to wash thoroughly and immediately, use an aerosol foam (if she has one) and see a doctor as soon as possible. Whatever happens, don't let her experiment with traditional do-it-yourself abortion remedies like bottles of gin and hot baths. They don't work, and can be dangerous.

Which form of contraception do women prefer?

It varies from woman to woman according to her tastes and experience. Once she finds a method she feels comfortable with, she is unlikely to experiment with others. In spite of the risks, most younger women choose to go on the Pill, and some special groups, such as sportswomen, who find their sexual rhythms a nuisance, prefer it because of its ability to suppress menstrual periods. But on the whole, IUD is probably the least obvious and harmful, provided she can find one that fits.

Which is the best form of contraception for sex?

Some couple prefer condoms and diaphragms because they can become a form of sex play in themselves. But in terms of natural freedom of sexual activity, without worries about health risks and pregnancy, vasectomy is probably the best for men and IUD for women.

CONCEPTION AND FERTILITY

How can I ensure conception? What is the best time and method?

When she starts her menstrual period, stop using any form of contraception but maintain your usual pattern of sexual activity. Then, provided you are both fertile, all you have to do is to enjoy deep vaginal intercourse – as deep as possible to give your sperm a fighting chance – on the thirteenth through fifteenth day of her sexual cycle, when she is most likely to be ovulating. There is no harm in letting yourselves go because a forceful ejaculation combined with good muscular spasm can get the sperm into the uterus in thirty seconds. If possible, withdraw about halfway through the ejaculation because the fluid from the prostate, which comes first, boosts the sperm while the last few ejaculations, from the seminal vesicles, may actually harm them.

If her temperature goes up during the twenty-four hours after intercourse you will know that your timing was right and there is a good chance that conception took place.

Is there a preferred position of intercourse for conception?

Any position which allows deep penetration, such as the woman squatting over you or lying underneath with her knees drawn up.

How does the previous use of contraception affect a woman's chances of conception?

All contraception should be stopped before you attempt to conceive. She should remove any IUD or diaphragm, and come off the Pill. It may take her body some time to adjust to its natural rhythms after stopping the Pill and this can affect conception by speeding up or delaying ovulation. Other forms of contraception have no lasting effect.

My partner and I have been trying to have a child for a long time, without success. What could be wrong and and what should we do?

The only way to find out what's the matter is for you and your partner to go to a family planning clinic or hospital for thorough tests. Many cases of infertility can be cured and the chances are that something can be done for you. Anxious couples in this position receive a sympathetic hearing and are offered confidential advice. Should either of you prove to be sterile, you will have the alternatives, such as artificial insemination or adoption, explained to you.

Is there a difference between sterility, infertility and and impotence?

Sterility means a permanent inability to conceive children.

Infertility is the temporary inability to do so, and falls into two categories – sexual performance that does not result in full ejaculation (*impotence*), and cases where the ejaculation is all right but the sperm themselves are too few or too weak to fertilize the egg. You will certainly know whether you can ejaculate, but there is no way to discover whether your sperm is fertile without microscopic analysis.

What can go wrong with sperm to make them infertile?

There can be too few of them (if the average count of about 250 million sperm per milliliter drops below about 50 million); too little seminal fluid (which fails to protect the sperm against the acids in the vagina); too much seminal fluid (which washes them out); or malformed sperm (which cannot swim far or fast enough).

Infertility can be caused by a wide range of factors including heredity, childhood diseases (or mumps when you are an adult), overheating the testicles (tight underwear), poor health or nutrition (especially lack of vitamins), smoking, drinking, stress, too long abstinence from sex (which causes more malformed sperm) and, in rare cases, exposure to radioactivity.

How can I tell if a child is mine?

If there is a choice between alternative "fathers," the only evidence which could be proved in court would be a blood type match or chromosome count. Neither of these will definitely establish that you *are* the father, but a different blood group from yours can prove that you are *not*. If you are still doubtful, you either accept her story (the woman usually has a good idea who it is) or wait till the child is old enough to recognize (though this, of course, is not reliable).

Advances in the science of genetic engineering and tissue-typing may soon make identification of the father possible.

What are "fertility drugs," and do they work?

It is hardly surprising that research into the contraceptive pill should have produced a parallel line of research into the opposite – a method of increasing the chances of conception. In fact, one of the first chemicals tried as a contraceptive, *clomiphene*, had the reverse effect, and is now on the market as a fertility drug. Sometimes these drugs fail to work but on other occasions they have resulted in widely publicized multiple births. Whether you see the reports as spectacular or grotesque depends on your point of view, but they point up the difficulty of judging the correct dosage of these highly unreliable chemicals.

Like the contraceptive pill, fertility drugs consist of chemicals which mimic the body's processes, but aim to increase, rather than prevent, ovulation. Some of them imitate the natural hormones which start ovulation, and others stimulate the pituitary gland in the base of the brain so that the hormones are manufactured normally. In the first type of drug (such as *pergonal*) the slightest miscalculation can release more than one egg, which is the cause of multiple births.

The long-term effects of these drugs have yet to be analyzed, but they are unlikely to be significant unless they are used repeatedly over a long period. In the meantime, although they are not a guarantee of fertility, they do offer many childless couples their only hope of parenthood.

PREGNANCY

Is there an easy way for us to check on her pregnancy?

The best way is the standard urine test, known as the HGG Test, carried out by clinics, mail-order laboratories or your own home kit. It consists of adding chemicals to a sample of her urine, takes only a few minutes and is 95 percent accurate after the fortieth day of a pregnancy.

If the test is positive she should have a clinical diagnosis between the sixth and tenth week to confirm the result. The doctor will check whether her uterus is enlarged and the cervix has turned the bluish color typical of pregnancy.

Can I tell if she is lying about the pregnancy?

Not for the first three months, until the uterus begins to expand beyond the pelvis and her stomach swells. She herself will probably know long before this, when she misses her periods and begins to experience the symptoms of hormonal changes such as morning sickness, enlarged and tender breasts and an increased appetite – not to mention the urine test she has almost certainly had done.

How long can I go on making love to a woman when she is pregnant?

If you love her you will leave the choice of sexual activity to her. In the early stages of pregnancy she can behave more or less normally, but she will probably show less interest in physical activity. This does not mean that she feels less in need of affection, and it may even be the moment when you discover the real difference between lovemaking and sex. The gentlest touch can carry a high sexual charge if it is meant.

If she wants it, there is no reason why you should not enjoy sex with each other (with care and consideration) until well into the pregnancy.

Can vaginal intercourse during pregnancy endanger the child?

Yes. Be careful and consult a doctor.

What about oral or anal sex, or masturbation?

Anal intercourse has the same effect on a pregnant womb as vaginal sex, but most other forms of activity and foreplay are open to you. If she wants to masturbate you or have oral sex, it is her choice.

Do the hormone changes affect her desire for sex?

The hormonal changes she undergoes affect her in different ways. During the first three months the imbalance may produce extreme changes of mood and an ambivalent attitude toward her pregnancy. Her body is now producing hormones to stop ovulation and the rest of the sexual cycle, and this may reduce the general level of her sexual desires. She may not react in the ways that you are used to, so make no assumptions about what she wants.

Is there any way of telling if the child is a boy or a girl?

If a cell sample is taken from the fetus or the fluid in the womb, as is done with tests for suspected genetic disease, it is possible to tell the sex of the child by a chromosome count. Apart from this test, and in spite of the increasingly accurate pictures taken by X-rays or ultra-sonography, you will still have to wait till the child is born to find out its sex.

How soon can I make love to her after the child is born?

As soon as she wants you, but don't expect it to happen immediately because her sexual interest has probably been reduced by the emotional upheaval and lowered estrogen levels. Apart from her natural soreness, she may suffer from muscular cramps and other physical discomfort, and for this reason doctors usually recommend waiting about six weeks after birth.

When you resume sexual activity, be careful about contraception. Her diaphragm will probably not fit any more, and she must not go back on the Pill if she is breast-feeding (though she might have a special Pill prescribed by her doctor), so it is best to use a condom with spermicides.

Does having a child affect her physiologically?

There is a steady loss of blood from the vagina for ten days, as the placenta and uterine lining break down. She will be very sore, her breasts may be swollen and painful and she may be suffering emotional moods as her hormone balance goes back to normal. Her cervix may be inflamed and it will take six weeks for her internal organs to return to their original size and position. It will be just as long before her menstruation resumes (this could take up to twenty-four weeks if she is breast-feeding), and ovulation does not begin again until at least twenty weeks after the birth.

As her regular cycle returns, her muscles regain their tone and her body gradually returns to normal. The only long-term effects may be a loss of shape to the breasts, which become fuller and more pendulous, and the possible presence of "stretch marks," like fine scars on her stomach and thighs.

Sexual Variations

Here are some of the common expressions of sexuality, from masturbation to homosexuality, defused of their more obvious myths and hang-ups. We have not gone into the more exotic activities such as sadomasochism, because we would either say too little or too much. If you have reached that stage, you probably know enough about yourself not to need our advice anyway. But if you are curious, still exploring, dreaming a little or just thinking about it, then read on. After all, the mind is an erogenous zone, and there's no harm in finding out about yourself.

MORALITY

**I can't help feeling guilty about anything but straight
sex. Aren't all these techniques and things immoral?**

Sex can be so many things, an obsession, a game, a ritual, duty,
chore, a form of self-discovery or religious experience. It can
express love, respect, friendship, status-seeking competition
and even hate. It is a language, something that can be learned,
misused, or even ignored – and sadly, more often than not,
suppressed. How can anything as wide as that, which adds so
much to human experience, be wrong?

"It is ethically right to do whatever heightens the pleasure
for yourself, so long as you do not harm anyone," said the
veteran New York therapist, Albert Ellis. "Indeed it may be
immoral not to practice helpful sexual techniques."

MASTURBATION

**Is there any truth in the old stories about masturbation
being dangerous to your physical or mental health?**

This is the oldest cliché in the book and complete nonsense. It
doesn't make you go blind, or lose your hair, or go to Hell. It
won't give you acne, or make you anemic. In fact, physiologi-
cally, it is indistinguishable from any other form of sexual
activity. All it will give you is pleasure and the opportunity to
explore your own sexuality. On the other hand, feeling guilty
about it or doing it in a hasty or furtive way can limit the
range of your sexual response with other people. When you
get into the habit of "getting it over" in five minutes, it can be
difficult to enjoy extended love play at other times.

Does masturbation make one tired and lackadaisical?

Not unless you are up all night doing it. In a sense, the reverse is true. It uses up similar energy as a brisk walk or jog, and is an excellent way of exercising your heart muscles.

Is masturbation a sign of immaturity that one should grow out of?

Learning to use and enjoy your own body is something you *grow into*. You have to be very foolish, or tired of life, to want to grow out of it.

Although few of them will admit it, 90 percent of men masturbate, with different frequencies and at different times, during their lives. There are certain groups of people who find it difficult or undesirable to form relationships with others for whom it becomes the only sexual outlet. The idea that it is "immature" is based on the fact that one of these deprived groups is comprised of teenagers who have not yet learned the social skills to make it any other way. Couples in their twenties and thirties are less likely to masturbate regularly. But self-sex becomes more common in late middle age and among the elderly, whose sexual desires can be as strong as ever, though our present social system denies them any outlet and even ridicules them for it.

Can the frequency of masturbation damage one's penis?

Frequency of any kind of sex, including masturbation, does no damage whatsoever. Kinsey reported men who masturbated six or seven times a day without the slightest effect on their health. But a habit which becomes compulsive leaves very little room for anything else in your life, and is usually a form of escape from boredom or unhappiness.

There is some evidence that a sudden change in sexual habits can upset the body's metabolism. In other words, suddenly stopping regular masturbation can be much worse than starting it in the first place.

At what age do boys start masturbating?

Anyone who has regular care of young children knows that a form of masturbation is common among boys from the age of four or five. Of course there is no possibility of orgasm and the sexual pleasure is not distinguished from other body sensations, but they seem to obtain real comfort from it.

Unfortunately, many people still hold the traditional Christian view that sex of any sort is incompatible with innocence, and feel it is their duty as parents to break these "dirty" habits. This attitude can set up life-long inhibitions which are passed on to the next generation in turn, in an unhappy circle.

Do women masturbate?

Yes, but apparently not as early or as often as men. There are a number of reasons for this. As children they do not have anything obvious to play with; they don't wake up with erections; the menstruation taboo sometimes puts them off having anything to do with it for a while; and generally they do not feel their bodies are their own property in the same way that men do. However, masturbation is the one way they can discover their own sexual desires and is considered an important therapy for women with problems such as frigidity.

For men, masturbation is a rough approximation of vaginal intercourse, but most women find it a completely different experience which requires a different frame of mind. Psychologically it is less of an "internal" experience of fantasies and closed eyes than it is for men, and many women prefer to make a ritual of it, with mirrors and soft lights so they can watch themselves.

I would like to watch my partner masturbate, but I feel it's wrong to do it with others. Isn't it something you should do alone?

If the taboo against masturbation is exaggerated, that against masturbation *with a partner* is even more extreme – and ridiculous. If it is possible for you to accept it as part of your sexual activity, and let your partner do likewise, it can be a voyage of discovery (and an education) for both of you.

SEX AIDS

Are dildos and vibrators just a way for women to masturbate?

It is a mistake to assume that dildos and vibrators are the same thing to a woman. They have quite different functions and it is only recently that commercial exploitation has killed one bird with two stones by combining them. The contradiction lies in the different ways we masturbate. Most men assume that women wish to simulate vaginal intercourse and the dildo was designed to reproduce the act of male penetration, whereas women generally prefer to masturbate by rubbing their clitoris or manipulating the whole vaginal area – which requires a different form of sex-aid altogether.

The penis-shaped probes called dildos or dildols have an ancient history in convents, harems, ritual deflorations, erotic art and metasex. They have been used in every recorded culture as power (virility) symbols, objects of worship, sexual devices for use with other women or men and, less effectively, to masturbate with. Vibration machines came into the picture when Masters and Johnson's famous sex report revealed that they could bring even frigid women to an orgasm, but these were *vibrating pads*, not buzzing plastic tubes. The sensation from a vibrating pad can be sexually stimulating for both men and women in many ways and, unlike dildos, a pad is not just a substitute for something else. With a little imagination a whole range of sex aids could be developed on the principle, but it is difficult to avoid the conclusion that the commercial vibrators now available are an example of men forcing their sexual imagery on women.

Do "love potions" and aphrodisiacs really work?

"Love potions" are drugs. It is difficult to think of them in this way when you consider their harmless ancestry in fairy stories and Shakespeare's plays, but they are, and before you try them you should be sure in your mind that you wouldn't rather let nature take its course.

Science has been unable to come up with the legendary potion which makes a specific person fall in love with you, although some drugs do exist which increase sexual desire in a general sense. However, most of them are unobtainable even with a prescription and none of them has anything to do with powdered rhino horn or shark's fin soup, or whatever traditional recipe you last had passed on to you. There are many drugs, including alcohol, which release inhibitions and have a significant effect on sexual encounters. There are also drugs which increase your sensitivity to touch and this can have much the same effect as an aphrodisiac. Marijuana and certain organic hallucinogens can heighten your awareness of your own body and intensify the sexual experience.

The truth is that a little imagination and boldness does the job better than any chemical cocktail. If you really want to extend your sexual activity glucose tablets will almost certainly give you more mileage than any commercial "aphrodisiac." It is necessary to use the word "almost," because anything which gives you confidence and belief in yourself will work wonders. People are capable of far more intense sexuality than most of them ever realize and all that is needed is a means of releasing them from unconscious inhibitions, ignorance and self-doubt. Which is why, when you come to think of it, the most powerful aphrodisiac in the world is someone else's desire for you.

There are lots of creams and ointments on sale as sex aids. What are they all for, and do they work?

No sex shop these days is complete without a drugstore of preparations promising to make your love life smoother, slower or better-smelling. They fall into three main groups: the cosmetic and toilet preparations, such as perfumes, powders and such exotica as tablets to "flavor" the taste of a vagina; the lubricants and oils, which may sometimes be necessary, but are usually just for fun; and the retardants which claim to prolong the pleasure.

Do the "retardants" really keep you going longer?

Retardants are a variety of creams and other applications which desensitize the nerve endings in your skin with a mild anesthetic. They won't help you keep an erection (that's up to you), but they will slow you down when you are very excited by slightly numbing the sensations. If you want to try them it is as well to remember that though they might give you a longer run, they also make it more difficult to get started if you apply them beforehand.

Of all the sex aids, the creams and lubricants are the easiest to incorporate into sex play and usually give the best value for money.

I've heard of "poppers" being used during sex. What are they?

"Poppers" are a drug, widely but often illegally available, which enormously heighten the sensations of sex without necessarily improving your physical performance. This is the vapor of a powerful stimulant called amyl nitrite. Small phials of the chemical in liquid form were originally manufactured for the use of heart patients in the form of glass tubes encased in fabric. When snapped in two they released the fumes, which is why they were first described as "poppers" by the people who discovered their other uses.

They are normally carried around in screw-top inhalers and used during sex because of their effect, especially during orgasm. The feeling is similar to a suspension of conscious thought and the release of instinctive passion from some primitive level of the brain which floods the body with over-powering physical sensation. Every touch and movement is so magnified that you lose yourself in your own body. The drug only works for a few minutes and repeated doses rapidly lose their effect. What you are doing, in effect, is to give yourself a mild heart attack. So while they can produce a transcendental sexual experience, they can be very, very dangerous.

Other stimulant drugs, such as amphetamine sulphate (speed) can have a remarkable effect on fantasies and "mental" sex, but act as such strong desensitizing agents that it can be difficult even to get an erection.

Are they dangerous?

The dangers of the indiscriminate use of powerful drugs are obvious. The risk of heart stimulants like "poppers" has been mentioned, but amphetamines are even more risky and can be addictive as well.

If you believe you have a right to choose what you put into your own body, and want to try them – be careful.

Most of the sex toys and attachments I've seen, such as

"ticklers," look uncomfortable and rather ridiculous. Are they worth trying?

If you are not turned on by the idea of them, there is no point in trying them to see if they work. You already know that they won't.

It all depends on what form of sexual activity you enjoy, and your attitude toward it. Some people have very few mental images or fantasies about sex. Others have an intensely serious attitude toward it and are embarrassed by the idea of sex-as-a-game. Or maybe they have a distaste for mechanical gadgets and see them as a substitute for the human body. For these people sex shops are bizarre and ludicrous.

But there are many people who find that the physical experience of sex is enriched by acting out their fantasies and letting their desires loose in wild daydreams. Ritual plays a large part in this, a defiance of taboos which makes the symbolic garments and devices in sex shops the direct descendants of the masks used in tribal societies.

What kinds of sex toys and equipment are available?

The simplest are the so-called "ticklers" – condoms which are shaped with protuberances or small knobs at the end, or with attachments such as rings or a fringe of bristles. These are designed to increase the stimulation for a woman during vaginal intercourse. They do little for the man except increase his ego, but if this is what you are after there are also ritual sheaths which extend the penis or show it off as a virility symbol. Then there are the mechanical substitutes for sex organs, such as dildos and inflatable "vaginas," and attachments which provide their own stimulation, like "cock rings" and the device, called Geisha spheres, for women, consisting of two small balls held in the vaginal cavity.

The main stock of any sex shop are the devices and garments

to help people act out individual fantasies. The range will be sadly limited and the prices high, but among the stereotypes you will usually find material for bondage fantasies, such as multiple belts and trusses, along with more overtly sado-masochistic material like whips and handcuffs. In among these, and in marked contrast, you will probably find the crotchless panties and frilly underwear of the "whore" fantasists. It all depends on which taboo you want to break, and the strength of your dreams. The person browsing through the crotchless panties is probably not interested in rubberware; and the guy asking about heavy ironware may be quite unmoved by transparent brassieres. It is a matter of taste.

I get excited looking at pornographic magazines and pictures. Is this unhealthy or immature?

Pornography was probably the original form of literature and almost as old as writing itself. No effort to suppress it has ever fully succeeded; nor should it. If you can stimulate your other emotions and appetites with pictures and descriptions (from cookery books and cartoons to thrillers and prayer books) there is no reason why you should not get excited by erotica and pornography.

There is an academic argument as to whether pornography is "real art," but it is certainly *not* unhealthy. The most thorough investigation of pornography yet carried out was probably the US Congressional Report in 1972, which was all but suppressed by Nixon's embarrassed administration because of its uncompromising conclusion that pornography was *not* harmful by any measurable medical or psychological standards. On the contrary, it was found to be beneficial in many ways, bringing some relief to frustrated and unhappy people.

Pornography is gradually becoming tolerated and even

legalized in many western countries, and nowhere has there been any evidence of "damage" to the generation who have now been exposed to it. In Denmark and Holland it was found that after the initial boom of commercial sexploitation, the sales and distribution leveled off at acceptable limits – and was even reflected in lower sex-crime statistics.

So if you prefer to have the images on the printed page rather than the back of your mind, or just want to try someones else's fantasies for a change, feel free. There's nothing wrong with it except that it is not as good as the real thing.

ORAL SEX

What is oral sex?

Oral sex involves any contact between the mouth and other erogenous areas, including the genitals. The lips and tongue are highly erotic and sensitive areas which have always played a part in lovemaking. Kissing the lips or other parts of the body such as the breasts, deep kissing in which the tongue is inserted in the other's mouth, the sucking of the penis (*fellatio*) or oral contact with the vagina (*cunnilingus*) are all common forms of sexual behavior. They can be used as foreplay prior to intercourse or as an intense sexual experience in themselves.

How common is fellatio and cunnilingus?

Kinsey's figures showed that 60 percent of men enjoy oral-genital contact at some time in their lives, with fellatio as the most common method. About 45 percent of his sample had experienced it in heterosexual circumstances, and it is a frequent form of homosexual intercourse.

However, Kinsey's report is now rather dated and sexual habits, especially the popularity of cunnilingus, appear to have changed since it was compiled. Only 16 percent of his sample admitted giving cunnilingus, but the 1977 survey by Pietropinto and Simenauer (*Beyond the Male Myth*, Times Books, 1977), indicated that 54.5 percent of men positively enjoy it, and only 22.8 percent disliked or never did it. "Far from being an exotic variation practiced by a few or some sort of special service," said the authors, "it is fast approaching intercourse itself as a universal sexual outlet."

I've heard of "deep throat," but what does it mean and are there other special techniques of fellatio?

Fellatio, sometimes referred to as "sucking off" or "giving head" is a form of lovemaking where experience counts, because a slight accidental bite can bring proceedings to a painful halt. But with a little practice it is possible to keep the teeth out of the way by relaxing the jaw muscles and opening the mouth wide. Again, there is no need to force the whole penis into your partner's mouth and choke her. Provided that the lower shaft is manipulated at the same time, it is only necessary to caress the head of the penis with lips and tongue for the full effect to be experienced.

But the ultimate technique, which has been called "deep throat," involves relaxing the muscles of the esophagus so that the head of the penis is literally "swallowed." In this way even a large penis can be taken to its full length and the sensitive glans is actually massaged by the throat muscles. It is a trick which has long been used by sword-swallowers and requires considerable self-control and practice, but the result can give intense pleasure to both partners.

My partner refuses to let me come in her mouth because she says it tastes bad. What is the taste? Can it be poisonous?

Unless she is one of the rare people with a skin allergy to semen, it will do her no harm and is certainly *not* poisonous. The taste, on the other hand, is a matter of personal preference.

While some people regard it as an act of intimacy to accept an ejaculation in the mouth and enjoy swallowing it, others are repelled by the very idea. As a rule, the more familiar you are with an activity, the less inhibited your response. It is an acquired taste, so there is no point in forcing the issue.

The taste of semen varies considerably from person to person, and for some reason it can acquire a flavor from food you have eaten recently, especially if it was spicy. If you have not ejaculated recently, it will be slightly sweeter because of the build-up of milk-sugar in the mixture; otherwise it has a more salty taste. Either way it is quite harmless.

She also says that she will get urine in her mouth. If it comes through the same passage can it really be hygienic?

Provided that neither of you have an infection, there is not the slightest danger. Your body takes care to ensure that the urine does not mix with the semen (which might otherwise damage the sperm) by sealing off the bladder with a double ring of muscles. But even if it did not, urine is not poisonous.

However, it is both hygienic and considerate to wash the genitals regularly, if only to prevent the smell of bacterial activity on sweat and the accumulation of smegma under the foreskin, which can make oral-genital sex distinctly unpleasant for your partner.

Do women really enjoy cunnilingus?

Pietropinto and Simenauer described it as "a potent turn-on for both partners. . . . Because of the direct gentle-but-intense clitoral stimulation received, even women who have difficulty reaching an orgasm through intercourse have easily attained climaxes through this activity." Certainly many women have claimed that it is the ultimate sexual pleasure and prefer it to any other form of sex. But this does not necessarily mean that your partner is one of them. There are many women who prefer more strenuous activity to the gentle pleasures of cunnilingus, so it is unwise to make assumptions. The only way to find out, is to find out.

I find myself put off by the taste and smell of a vagina, especially during a woman's period. Is this usual?

You are not alone in this. The Pietropinto and Simenauer survey showed that about 25 percent of men rated odors and discharge as the "most unpleasant aspect of sex," second only to an unresponsive partner, and their sample showed a strong bias in favor of hygiene in other questions. As much as 70 percent found their sexual pleasure reduced during their partner's period.

Sex has many acquired tastes and smells and it is natural that they seem strange at first. But you are not born liking (or disliking) them and they only become emotionally charged by association with the pleasures (or unpleasantness) involved.

Both my partner and I enjoy oral sex, but her contraceptive jelly tastes awful. What can we do about it?

If cunnilingus forms a regular part of your lovemaking, it might be better to change your form of contraception. Or acquire a taste for it. Alternatively, if you want to go that far, it is possible to buy special tablets from sex-aid shops which "flavor" the vaginal passage – or you might experiment on your own with something from the kitchen cabinet!

ANAL SEX

What do people get out of anal sex? I find the whole idea disgusting.

Anal sex is certainly illegal in many states (which is as silly as legislating for any other sexual position), but if you find it disgusting you are in a minority. With most men and women, it comes second only to oral sex as the main variation. After all, it is not so different from the usual rear entry position for vaginal intercourse and in some circumstances, with obese people or pregnant women, it can be easier. The experience is much the same as vaginal sex except that the penis is gripped more tightly and, since the rectum is a larger cavity, deep penetration is more comfortable.

There is no denying that the anus is sensitive – just feel it. In fact, it is a highly erogenous zone in both sexes.

Isn't it unhygienic?

Of the various types of sexual activity, the most unhygienic is kissing. Compared with that, anal sex is perfectly safe, providing you wash regularly and neither of you has VD. Although the lower end of the intestines contains a bacteria (eschericia coli or e. coli) which can infect other parts of the body, there is no statistical evidence to connect anal intercourse with infections of the penis.

Can it damage the anus?

Rough treatment can damage any sexual organ and the sphincter muscle of the anus can certainly be damaged if it is forced. There is no need for that, but if the sphincter is damaged or torn, it must be treated like any other wound, and if it doesn't clear up you should consult a doctor.

Is there a special technique?

Some people find it difficult to relax enough for anal intercourse. We are taught as babies to tighten and restrain the
sphincter muscles so that the "pulling in" reflex is almost
instinctive. But in order to receive an object like a penis one
must relax the muscles by "pushing out."

Do that, take it gently (with a little lubricant), and it's easy.

I often have a strong desire to urinate before or after sex. Is there a reason for this?

There could be several. Nervousness and excitement, for
instance, can both be accompanied by an urgent need to find
the bathroom. Then there is the biological fact that when you
get an erection your bladder is automatically shut off by
sphincter muscles. This tends to compress it slightly, making
it feel fuller than it is; and by the same token it might fill up
while you are enjoying yourself and be in need of release
afterward. Or maybe you just equate urination with sexual
activity. Whatever the reason, it is nothing to worry about.

I find the idea of urination sexually exciting. Is there something wrong with me?

No – except that you need to ask such questions. The same
childhood taboos that apply to excretion also apply to
urination. If you enjoyed being "naughty" then, you probably will now. And if your prejudices were reinforced as you
grew older you will find the idea even more disgusting now.
In some people this fear and distaste unfortunately come to
include the whole genital area and, as a result, sex in general.

At a simple, practical level, this is nonsense. Try putting it
the other way around. If sex is fun, why shouldn't urination

be? The rest of the animal kingdom is uninhibited enough about it, and so are many human beings. Even without the evidence of numerous letters to every "contact" magazine, sexologists are well aware of how widespread the practice is. It is not unusual for people to be turned on by the thought of urinating on each other, or letting go during vaginal intercourse (especially for the man when the woman does it), or simply watching someone do it. Even the drinking of urine (*urolagnia*) is harmless.

Urine, after all, is mainly water – just ordinary water which contains, in weak solution, a few surplus body salts and the materials which our bodies cannot metabolize (urea, uric acid and creatinine), together with coloring matter. No one is quite sure what this yellow coloring (*urochrome*) is, but it seems to be quite harmless. Urine has only a faint smell and taste. The strong smell of ammonia often associated with it only develops later as a result of bacterial action.

One word of warning, however, to those who want to realize their fantasies. It is very difficult to urinate with an erection. Except, paradoxically, with those leaden early-morning erections which won't go down until you've sprayed half the bathroom.

Homosexuality

Most of the questions in this book are those asked by heterosexuals, about themselves, about women in general and their female partners in particular. But as many as a third of our readers will have had a sexual experience with their own sex at some time in their lives. Whatever the law may say in your part of the world (and it varies in contradictory confusion from one place to another), homosexuality is here to stay. So we make no apology for including it as a normal and valid sexual experience.

ATTITUDES

I think I might be homosexual, but how can I tell?

Try not to make up your mind too soon. It is perfectly possible for you to have a deep emotional feeling for another man without being "gay," or you may just be discovering a bisexual aspect of your personality. But if you find yourself strongly attracted to other men, if they figure in your fantasies and you seek out physical contact with them, then the chances are that you have a predominantly homosexual nature. In the final result, it is something that only you can decide.

What does that make me?

There is no need to panic. What it does *not* make you is a member of a sinful, neurotic, freakish minority. You can forget the cliches and dirty jokes. There are as many as 200 million homosexuals in the world – the vast majority of them living full, satisfactory and useful lives. It would be impossible to identify most of them by physical characteristics, mannerisms or dress, although increasing numbers of them are openly declaring their sexuality. They are as capable of love and can achieve as full sexual satisfaction as heterosexuals. In other words, they are just as responsible, depraved, happy, unhappy, criminal, eccentric or normal as anyone else.

What proportion of society is homosexual?

Strangely enough, very few surveys have been attempted to establish this simple fact. Many authors and sociologists have made private assessments, but none of the major sexual studies carried out in the last few years is entirely convincing or even agrees with another. The Pietropinto and Simenauer survey had a reactionary anti-homosexual bias, Shere Hite's report was radical feminist and pro-lesbian, the Hunt study and Master and Johnson are inadequate in other respects and only Kinsey produced a half-way valid set of figures.

Trying to be as objective as possible, it seems likely that in the USA and other western industrialized countries, up to 5 percent of people are exclusively homosexual, 10 percent to 15 percent have sought out bisexual experiences in adult life and about a third of the whole population has had at least one homosexual experience to orgasm between adolescence and old age.

These figures are based on a western Anglo-Saxon culture which is intensely anti-erotic, and if it were not for the prejudice and hypocrisy of our society the figures would probably be much higher. In many countries, especially in the Middle and Far East, homosexuality is publicly accepted, with its own social conventions.

The figures tend to show that sexuality is a continuous spectrum with exclusive single-sex attraction at either end. The ideal balance may well be half-way along. After all, love is difficult enough to find without excluding half the race.

Is homosexuality more common in any particular social group?

No. Generally speaking it occurs in all social groups, although certain conventions may make it easier to express (in the armed forces, prison or any single-sex society) or more difficult (in narrow-minded, small-town communities, for instance). There are two qualifications to this. The Pietropinto and Simenauer survey showed a tendency for poorer and less educated groups to be more conservative and inhibited about sex; and it is common for young "gays" to want to escape the restrictions of family life, so there is a preponderance of them living in big cities, where there are better facilities for meeting each other.

Why is the word "gay" used to describe homosexuals?

Because it is the first, and only, name they have chosen for themselves. The word "homosexuality" is still acceptable and says what it means (homo means "same," incidentally, not "male") but it is a cold technical term for a whole way of life. In the past the only alternative has been insulting slang which has varied from place to place, but always carried the same message of derision. So when the homosexual political movements formed in the early 1970s, they hijacked the word "gay" from the English dictionary to replace the jeers and taunts. In the same way as the blacks or the women's movement, the "largest minority" as it has been called, demand the right to choose what they are called. Whatever "gay" once meant, with or without invested commas, it now means homosexual.

Who does what and with which and to whom?

There is no mystery about gay sexual activity because, except for the substitution of anal for vaginal intercourse, it is no different from heterosexual activity. It covers the same variations, including fellatio and mutual masturbation. As with heterosexual activity, it is responsive foreplay, sensitivity to the other's sexual arousal and the feelings which are expressed, which matter.

But heterosexual intercourse, male gay sex and lesbianism all show distinct psychological differences. The pattern of heterosexuality is established by the fact that there are two types of people involved who are biologically and emotionally different. This sets up all sorts of tensions and attractions which are alien to gay sex, where the responses and desires are the same for each person. A woman can guess at what a man feels as he is building up to an orgasm, she may even empathize

122

with him, but she can never actually *know* in the same way as another man. This mutuality leads to different sexual expression among men and women. Male gays tend to have more muscular, rhythmic, orgasm-oriented, wrestling sex, based on active movement and exploiting their familiarity with the male body. Lesbians, on the other hand, often have more gentle but emotionally more intense relationships, with extensive manipulation but little physical activity or penetration.

Is it true that homosexuals are promiscuous?

Some people have described the gay lifestyle as promiscuous, and the opportunity, or rather choice, does exist. But this only puts the responsibility on each individual to work out his own morality.

Perhaps the most distinctive characteristic of gay activity is that it is free of all social conventions which condition the relationships between men and women. There are no age or class barriers for instance. There are no social pressures such as marriage to hold unsuccessful relationships together. In fact, there are many which work in the opposite direction. But, in spite of this, long-term relationships do evolve, though it is common for gays to have a much wider sexual experience than a heterosexual of the same age. Paradoxically, because it is a mainly "underground" activity, it is much easier for a gay to find sexual partners. Every reasonable size town and city has established rendezvous, and these are listed in numerous directories and guides. But surprisingly enough, many of these bars and clubs and steam baths exist more for the emotional companionship of other gays than as places to pick people up.

Surely the purpose of marriage is to have children. How can homosexuals have a permanent

relationship without them?

The fact that there are no children is often regarded as a tragic aspect of being gay, though it does have the advantage of giving each partner a clearer focus for their emotions. But many gays, especially lesbians, feel the absence of children deeply, and pressure groups are trying to amend existing legislation to allow them to adopt children. There are arguments for and against this, but the discussion is usually drowned out by the same hysteria and prejudice which affects every aspect of homosexuality.

What about the homosexual's reputation for interfering with children?

This widespread myth is the exact reverse of the truth.

A strong emotional attraction toward children is medically classified as *pedophilia*, and occurs across all the boundaries of sex and age. Since it is as common among heterosexuals as homosexuals, young girls are in far greater danger from "straight" pedophiles than young boys are from gays. The association with "dirty old men" is just as inaccurate. The overwhelming majority of sexual assaults on children occur within the home and are committed by males under twenty-five years old.

In spite of the fierce social taboo against pedophilia, there is little evidence that it does serious harm to the children and many cultures have deliberately allowed for the expression of children's sexuality. The real damage is done by the violence which sometimes accompanies the assault and by the hysterical reaction of the child's parents. If these become associated in the child's mind with the sexual element it can seriously inhibit its adult life.

Is it true that homosexuals can be recognized by

physical differences such as wide hips?

Physical characteristics have nothing to do with sexual inclination. Unless a gay wants you to know, there is no way that you will recognize him. The "sure signs" of homosexuality are about as bizarre as a medieval catalog of ways to recognize witches, and about as effective. The very fact that there is no identifiable difference is the main problem gays have in forming a coherent social unit. This is why the radical liberation movement makes a point of wearing signs and badges proclaiming who they are and criticize the "closet queens" who pass for heterosexuals.

Then how do homosexuals recognize and meet each other?

A few have the courage to deliberately express the feminine elements in their character with clothes and mannerisms, but the majority simply go to the places where other homosexuals go – and take a chance. If they want to get to know someone they use exactly the same approaches and body language as a heterosexual male would use in similar circumstances with a woman.

I am confused by such terms as "transsexual" and "transvestite." Are they forms of homosexuality?

These terms are often confused because of their association with the wearing of women's clothes by men, but they are quite different phenomena and neither is directly connected with homosexuality.

Transvestites are people who achieve sexual satisfaction by wearing the more distinctive clothes of the opposite sex. Although homosexuals sometimes dress like this to express the feminine element in their personality, it is just as likely to be

125

an expression of *desire for* the opposite sex. Transvestism probably occurs more often within marriage than outside it.

Transsexuals on the other hand, are people who believe that sexually and psychologically they *should be* the opposite sex. They feel trapped inside the wrong biological body and sometimes go so far as to seek sex-change surgery to correct it. Transsexual men often adopt a totally female lifestyle, wearing women's clothing, not for sexual pleasure, but because anything else feels unnatural. They are no more homosexual than transvestites, because they want to relate to men as *women*, not as other men. They specifically want to be the opposite sex, rather than taking pleasure in being the same.

What is "gay liberation"?

Although there have been a number of discrete homosexual organizations in the past, such as the US Mattachine Society, it is usually agreed that the gay liberation movement emerged as a result of the Christopher Street riots in 1969, when a large proportion of the homosexual population of New York's Greenwich Village took a stand against police harrassment, exploitation and underworld extortion. The GLF (Gay Liberation Front) and the GAA (Gay Activist Alliance) were formed as a result, and the movement rapidly spread to Europe.

The movement, on both sides of the Atlantic, now covers a wide range of organizations from pressure groups and telephone counseling services to the wildest street politics. What they have in common is a belief in themselves, the rejection of the old definitions of "sickness" and "criminality" and a determination to live their lives as openly and honestly as anyone else. Many of these organizations, such as CHE in Britain, campaign against discriminatory laws, while the more radical groups go still further with experiments in communal living, association with existing (usually left-wing) political parties and, as in the case of FUORI in Italy and FAHR in France, even resort to overt guerrilla action against the establishment.

CAUSES

What causes homosexuality?

There has been a fierce (but almost completely uninformed) debate about this for many years. There is still very little evidence and no one really knows the answer, but there are three main theories.

The genetic theory is that a basic sexual inclination, probably based on the balance of hormones, is inherited from the parents and that this is expressed or brought out in childhood.

The psychological theory, which is much thought of by school teachers and Freudian analysts, is that the person's psychological "growth" from the autoeroticism of babies to the heterosexuality of adults gets stuck at an intervening stage of homosexuality.

The more recent behaviorist theory is that one is born with an indiscriminate sexuality which is conditioned to a certain pattern when one is very young and that this can be reinforced or modified during childhood. All the theories agree that by adolescence a person's sexuality is more or less established as a fundamental part of their psychology.

The genetic explanation has always been popular among gays themselves because it provides the clear-cut answer— "I was born that way," but it is increasingly discounted for lack of evidence. Extensive experiments with hormones have shown that although they alter the intensity of the sexual drive they do nothing to alter its direction.

The psychological theory has had a better run, but again

there is little evidence. In this case, though, there are any number of explanations, usually expressed in Freudian terms. Family life is seen as a traumatic minefield for a child and the young homosexual is trapped in an elaborate scenario of symbols and double meanings, peopled with characters from Greek mythology. One can take one's choice from a dominant mother and absent father, or weak mother and hero-worshipped father, or no parents at all and identification with a single-sex peer group – or whatever happens to fit the evidence.

"My mother made me a homosexual," runs the old gay joke. "If I send her some wool," comes the reply, "would she make me one too?"

The behaviorist theory is probably the most widely accepted. A baby, after all, has to learn almost every aspect of its behavior, from the task of focusing its eyes to discovering who and what it is. It even has to learn to learn. So it is hardly surprising that a part of this process should be learning how and whom to love.

TREATMENT

Can homosexuality be cured?

Since there is no illness or recognized standard of health, the word "cure" has very little meaning. But over the years there have been many attempts to redirect or suppress sexual conduct that did not conform to the social code of the time. The methods usually relied on sanctions, from cold baths to castration and even capital punishment, but they had little effect on human nature. Nowadays, however, with hormones, mood-altering drugs and aversion therapy, a crude form of psychological surgery is possible. It is difficult to control the side effects (which can be horrendous) or to predict the outcome, so people agree to it only under duress or in despair.

The chemotherapy technique involves the use of hormones and drugs to suppress all sexual desires, like a form of lobotomy. But the main technique, now used in clinics and hospitals around the world, is a brainwashing system called *aversion therapy*.

This consists of subconscious "teaching" to reprogram deeply ingrained habits or emotions. The patient is exposed to a number of stimuli, some of which are associated with his "problem," and when he responds to the "bad" images or sensations he is treated to electric shocks or nausea-inducing drugs. A homosexual, for instance, might be shown a succession of male and female pornography and "punished" over and over again at the appropriate image, until a new behavior pattern is forced into his subconscious.

At a simple level, aversion therapy has had some success in curing kleptomaniacs and compulsive gamblers, but when it comes to altering basic emotions, the patient's entire personality is at risk. At best it seems to repress the fundamental sex drive by inducing an acute guilt complex, leaving the patient socially "cured" but psychologically maimed.

Aversion therapy has sinister possibilities. Anyone who thinks that the Thought Police in George Orwell's *1984* are a sick fantasy, might consider this. In 1972, at Cuelvo in Spain, the Franco regime opened a concentration camp to which all homosexual prisoners were automatically remanded – the function of which was to carry out extensive and secret experiments in aversion therapy. The prisoners were condemned to indefinite sentences, put through appalling torture and were not released until they had been "certified" as heterosexual.

Venereal Disease

The first time you catch VD can be a humiliating experience – until you see how many people there are in the VD clinic and realize that you have one of the most common diseases in the world.

If you associate that initial shame and disgust with the lovemaking which preceded it, it could make your future a sour and unhappy prospect. The only moral issue about VD is to get it fixed as soon as possible, and the only thing you should feel guilty about is passing it on to someone else.

VD is not a reflection on sexual relationships, any more than breathing is responsible for influenza. As a wise physician once put it, "It's better to have a positive Wasserman test than never to have loved at all."

What is VD?

VD, or *venereal disease*, is not a specific complaint but a whole variety of different contagious diseases. About all that they have in common is the fact that they all flourish in the warm moist environment of body orifices such as the penis, vagina, rectum and mouth. Like all contagious diseases, they are passed from one person to another by physical contact and since these parts of the body usually only come in contact during sexual activity, they are described as venereal.

Some of them have been around since the beginning of history, but they really took hold in Europe in the early sixteenth century after Columbus' sailors are said to have brought syphilis back with them from the New World. It spread widely through the urban developments of the Industrial Revolution and since World War II there has been an even bigger boost, which has multiplied the incidence of the disease three or four times over. Nowadays it has reached epidemic proportions and is virtually out of control in many western countries. This has mainly been due to the combination of two social factors – freedom of movement and more liberated sexual attitudes on one hand, and the persisting guilt and embarrassment still attached to them, which discourages people from seeking immediate medical attention, on the other. VD is not the "wages of sin," nor an act of God, nor even a social disaster. It is no "dirtier" than any other disease and, but for this hangover from Victorian morality, it could be reduced or eliminated.

VD can be caused by bacteria or virus infections of different kinds. Most forms are easily cured, although some, particularly when there has been repeated infections, may require lengthy treatment. Some are no more than a painful inconvenience, while others, if they find their way into the central nervous system, can prove fatal.

What are the main forms of VD?

The worst is *syphilis*, the most common is *gonorrhea*, and there is a group of relatively mild but painful complaints called NSU, or *non-specific urethritis*. These are the main forms, but there are a number of comparatively rare venereal infections, usually only found in the tropics, such as *chancre*, *lympho-granuloma venereum* and *granuloma inguinale*. Finally, the genital area can also be infected by common skin disorders like warts, cold sores and lice, and these are sometimes classified as venereal diseases.

What should I do if I think I might have VD?

If you think (or even *suspect*) that you might have VD, seek medical help immediately from your family physician. Or if that is too embarrassing, from your firm's doctor, or local hospital, or anyone who can direct you to the nearest VD clinic. The clinics are designed to reduce your embarrassment to the minimum, and you will find them sympathetic, direct and unshockable.

What happens when you go to a VD clinic?

You will probably have a blood sample taken for a Wasserman (or similar) test, smears of any discharge you may have will be put under a microscope, and you will probably be asked for a sample of your urine for analysis. When these have been checked you will most likely be given a shot or two of anti-biotics, which will eradicate your symptoms in a few days. It is as simple as that.

After treatment you may be interviewed by a VD investi-gator, in order to track down your contacts. This is not an invasion of privacy, nor is the investigator just nosy. Your personal information will be kept confidential throughout. It is as much in your own interest as anyone else's to prevent the disease spreading and avoid reinfection. After all, it could be you who is being reinfected.

Remember that treatment and prevention of VD is an act of love.

What are the symptoms I should look out for?

Later stages of the diseases can have different symptoms, but these are usually the first to appear.

Discomfort in the penis. You should notice especially a burning sensation while urinating and the presence of a thick yellow-green discharge, along with painful erections. This can be either gonorrhea or NSU and requires laboratory analysis of a smear to decide which it is. With some forms of NSU the tip of the penis can be blocked with dried pus, and there may be blood in the urine.

Sores on the penis or genital area. There are at least four venereal diseases that produce sores in the early stages and laboratory tests are needed to distinguish between them. Syphilis usually produces a firm round or oval sore, about a $\frac{1}{2}$ inch across, which oozes a colorless fluid; chancre produces a group of elongated soft sores; lymphogranuloma venereum, a small blister or ulcer; and granuloma inquinale, bright red painless spots. If you have any sort of sore in the genital area, treat it as a symptom of VD.

Swollen glands. These usually appear around the genitals after the initial signs. They tend to occur in the top of the thigh, but in the case of NSU the testicles may also be swollen and tender.

Any one of these symptoms needs immediate attention. They may disappear of their own accord after a few weeks, but don't be misled by this. You still have the disease, but it is now in a quiescent, and more dangerous, form.

What is syphilis?

Syphilis, also known as "the pox" or "scab," is the most dangerous of venereal diseases because it goes through a number of quiet phases when nothing appears to be wrong with you. But, unlike other forms of VD, it inevitably spreads through the body if it is not treated, and eventually it will attack the heart and nervous system with crippling or fatal results. It also has the unpleasant characteristic of being passed on genetically.

The disease is caused by small spiral-shaped bacteria called *spirochetes*, which thrive in the warm passages of the genital organs and mouth, and are transmitted by contact with the affected part. Because it can be inherited from an infected mother, it can also appear, apparently spontaneously, years later.

The thousand or so bacteria you pick up on infection take about three weeks of incubation to multiply to two hundred million, and start making their presence felt. The first symptoms, suppurating sores and a slight swelling in the groin, will clear up in another few weeks. The bacteria are now moving out of the genital area into your body and soon a new set of symptoms will appear. There will be headaches, loss of appetite and fevers, accompanied by a dark red rash on the backs of your legs, the front of your arms and other parts of the body, together with swollen lymph glands. There is no itching, but there may be breaks in the skin. At the same time there may be loss of hair and sores on the mouth and genitals. Although these symptoms will also disappear in a few months, it is vital to have them treated, because when the third, or tertiary, symptoms occur it may be too late.

Tertiary symptoms can remain dormant for up to fifty years, though they sometimes follow in a matter of months. About a third of all those who have not yet been treated will develop them. They include crippling ulcers and lesions on bones and joints, blindness, paralysis, insanity and death.

What is the cure for syphilis?

Syphilis can be difficult to diagnose, because the early symptoms are often so mild, and it may take several laboratory tests to confirm its presence. In the first and second stages it can be completely cured by the use of penicillin and other antibiotics. Even in the tertiary stage the disease can sometimes be halted, although the existing damage would be irreversible.

What is gonorrhea?

Gonorrhea, sometimes refered to as "the clap," is a bacterial infection which has spread rapidly over the last few years. This is partly because the symptoms in women can be so slight that they do not even know they have it. But whatever the reason, it is now the second most frequent disease after the common cold and there is a strong possibility that you may have it at some time in your life. Unlike syphilis, it tends to be localized in your body, although it can cause arthritis of the joints in the later stages. It is caught by close body contact or sexual activity, though less often from oral contact than syphilis.

The incubation period is usually less than a week, though it can be longer, and the early symptoms are a burning pain and discharge from the penis. This can lead to abcesses within the urethra which make urination difficult and painful. The glands, especially the testicles, can become hard and swollen.

Gonorrhea can infect the rectum during anal intercourse and the symptoms are a similar discharge of yellowish fluid, soreness, itching and severe pain when defecating. This type can occur without any symptoms around the penis.

In the rarer cases of gonorrhea in the mouth, the symptoms are milder and often mistaken for a throat infection.

What is the cure for gonorrhea?

Gonorrhea is cured by penicillin and antibiotics. Certain strains are, however, now becoming resistant to these, and an ominous new strain has recently emerged which eludes medical treatment by breeding very fast. So it may be necessary to have a variety or combination of antibiotics. During treatment for this and all forms of VD, it is advisable to refrain from alcohol and masturbation. And, of course, from sexual intercourse.

What is NSU?

Non-specific urethritis is a cover name for a variety of diseases and infections with no detectable cause. Some might be due to unidentified micro-organisms and others to an imbalance in your own body chemistry. It is a very common form of VD, and unlike the others it is not necessarily transmitted by sexual activity. If you catch NSU it may have nothing to do with your partners, because it is possible for two people who were otherwise virgins to develop symptoms because of a chemical reaction against each other's hormones. It can also occur if you change your sexual habits too abruptly. Either way, it usually disappears after a few days when your metabolism has adjusted itself.

The symptoms are similar to those of gonorrhea. If they are not treated there is a one percent chance of developing a secondary stage, called *Reiter's disease*. This produces more severe symptoms including ulcers, skin rashes and arthritis.

What about the tropical forms of VD?

It must be stressed that these exotic forms of VD are comparatively rare, and unless you are visiting foreign ports you are unlikely ever to come across them. The ones previously mentioned were:

Chancre. These are "soft sores," which are caused by a rod-shaped bacterium which incubates for between three and five days. Either sex can carry the disease without symptoms, but when they appear they include ulcers on the penis and painfully swollen glands. The treatment is by antibiotics.

Lymphogranuloma venereum. This is another bacterial infection which is usually caught from sexual partners, although in some cases it can be picked up from infected bedding. It produces genital blisters after five to twenty-one days incubation, and there may be internal complications later on. It is also treated by antibiotics.

Granuloma inguinale. This is a bacterial infection which, once again, is normally caught through sexual activity. The symptoms are pimples which grow into a painless, raised area, a bright beefy red in color. Once again, it is treated with antibiotics.

Do women have the same symptoms of VD?

The symptoms are generally similar to those in men. There can be sores and rashes around the genital area, unusual vaginal discharge, swollen glands and pain when urinating, as well as during intercourse and menstruation. They tend to be milder and less obvious in the early stages, because sores in the vagina are less noticeable than sores on the penis. The diseases also develop in much the same way, except in the case of gonorrhea.

Gonorrhea in women has a longer incubation period, and the symptoms can amount to no more than a small vaginal discharge. This not only makes them more dangerous as carriers of the disease, it also puts them at greater risk because they are less likely to obtain medical treatment. The risk is considerable, because although the early symptoms are mild, the later ones are severe. If left untreated, the disease can cause swollen glands around the vagina, and spread to the rectum because the openings are so close. Eventually it can affect internal organs causing sickness, pain and possible sterility. In the case of pregnant women it can result in the death of both mother and fetus.

I don't believe the old stories about catching it from lavatory seats, but is it possible to get VD any other way than sex?

The usual answer to this is no, because the germs which cause VD rapidly die outside the warm body environment. But there is a recent theory that gonorrhea might be carried by pubic lice, in which case the "old story" may be true.

There are a few, rare ways in which it can be caught apart from sexual activity. Dentists, for instance, have been known to catch syphilis from infected mouths, and the bacteria which cause lymphogranuloma venereum can survive outside the human body. But the overwhelming majority of VD cases are contracted by kissing (which doesn't necessarily have to be sexual, when you think about it) or by some other form of intimate body contact.

Is it true that you can take antibiotics after sex to protect you from VD?

It is true that penicillin tablets taken just before or after sexual intercourse will help to protect you from VD, although it is by no means guaranteed. But while an anti-VD tablet is feasible, and can even be obtained at some clinics, the effects could be disastrous. The more penicillin you use, the more chance there is of developing an allergy to it – and a bad penicillin reaction can be worse than gonorrhea. At the same time, bacteria such as gonorrhea rapidly become resistant to antibiotics, and if everyone took these pills, sooner or later there would be no cure for the disease. The combination of unnecessarily overdosing yourself at the same time as you are breeding resistant bacteria makes it a thoroughly anti-social idea. The best way to combat the disease is not by worrying about it beforehand, but by owning up quickly and fully when you get it.

Why isn't there a permanent cure for VD, such as a vaccine?

When vaccines have all but eliminated diseases like polio, it may seem surprising that none has been developed against VD. But there are reasons for this, quite apart from the storm of protest which would be raised by the "guardians" of public morality. In the case of syphilis, the initial blood tests are the only positive way of identifying the disease, and vaccines would tend to produce the same results as the disease itself. To deprive doctors of this diagnostic test would only help to spread the disease. In the case of gonorrhea, if a vaccine were developed it would be similar to that for cholera, which is only effective for six months at a time. It would be difficult to know whether you were properly protected at any given time, and would also put an enormous strain on the medical services.

Does this mean that there are no preventive measures that I can take?

Although prevention, as always, is better than cure, in the case of VD it is a lot more difficult.

One way is to abstain from sex, but this is going a little too far – and, anyway, it is no protection against NSU and may cause prostate trouble. The next best way is probably to make sure you know when you are taking chances. And not only when you are taking them, but where, and with whom. There is no reliable guideline to this except experience. There are people who sleep around and those who don't. The former are more likely to have VD, but also more likely to be honest with themselves and open with you about it. The latter are less likely to have it, but more likely to be embarrassed about telling anyone. Of course, you can always look for symptoms on your partner. If it has got to that stage in your friendship, there is no harm in looking anyway.

When it comes down to it, there are a few practical precautions which will improve your chances, even if they don't actually protect you. The most effective of these is to use a condom and spermicidal foam during sexual intercourse. Then, in rapidly descending order of reliability, there are: the use of vaginal antiseptics and suppositories; urinating immediately after intercourse; and washing thoroughly before and after.

Male Health Problems

There are such things as "men's diseases." Just as there are certain complaints which only affect women, there are others which only affect men. Sometimes the distinction results from our anatomy. Women, for instance, only have a rudimentary prostate gland, so there is a whole range of prostate conditions that apply exclusively to men. Then there are other biological differences which mean that we are more likely to suffer complaints like some types of hernias. But these are not the only ones. The inherited diseases of hemophilia and muscular dystrophy are primarily male afflictions. Color blindness is far more common in men than women. About 90 percent of sufferers from peptic ulcers are men, and so are 95 percent of cases of gout.

It is not clear why this should be so, but certain clues are coming to light. It seems that women are more likely to develop some of these illnesses – gout and ulcers, for instance – after the menopause. The female sex hormone, estrogen, stops being produced at this time, so it has been suggested that it may have some preventative role. Many of these complaints are hereditary (gout, particularly, is often passed down through families), which seems to support the hormone theory. But this is not always the case and the full mechanism of these diseases has yet to be worked out.

HEMORRHOIDS

What are hemorrhoids?

Hemorrhoids, or "piles," are a complaint suffered by most men at some time or another, especially as they get older. They consist of enlarged blood vessels, rather like varicose veins, which produce swellings in the lining of the anus. They are usually caused by acute constipation, over-straining during excretion, by loss of muscle tone or, occasionally, by anal intercourse. The symptoms are pain and sometimes slight bleeding from the anus, particularly during excretion. The piles are usually just inside the anus, but if they protrude beyond it they can be painfully squeezed by the sphincter muscles – a condition known as *strangulation.*

The discomfort and burning sensations hardly need to be described to anyone who has experienced them, but piles are not dangerous and can be treated immediately with ointments and suppositories available at any drugstore. Unfortunately, once one has had piles, they are liable to recur; and if they are left untreated they may ultimately need surgical treatment.

ULCERS

What are peptic ulcers?

There are two kinds of *peptic ulcers*: sores on the lining of the stomach, which are known as *gastric ulcers,* or in the intestine just below the stomach, called *duodenal ulcers.* Gastric ulcers are much less common (10–20 percent of peptic ulcer cases).

If your appetite is affected, you feel like vomiting and have pains in the upper abdomen between half and hour and two hours after meals, you may well have a gastric ulcer. If the pains occur between two and two and a half hours after meals, while your appetite remains healthy and eating may even soothe the pain, then the ulcer is probably in the duodenum. In both cases the pain is usually worse on an empty stomach and the area is tender to touch.

In severe cases the ulcer can penetrate a blood vessel and cause hemorrhaging, or it can obstruct the passage of food, causing muscular spasms and swelling. If the ulcer "perforates," or works its way right through the stomach wall, the digestive juices burst through into the body cavity and can result in peritonitis. This is an extremely serious condition which requires immediate surgery.

What causes them?

Ulcers are still something of a mystery. It is thought that they start with a small cut or tear in the stomach lining, and that this is then aggravated by the digestive juices – a matter of literally "eating yourself up." But this does not explain why 90 percent of sufferers are men, or why the ulcer, instead of spreading like any other sore, covers only a small area while drilling straight down into the stomach lining. Hereditary factors and hormone balances are thought to be involved, and there seems to be a bias against people with blood group "O." It is known that stress, excessive drinking and rich food all aggravate the condition.

What is the treatment?

Mild ulcers usually clear up with a regime of rest, antacids and frequent bland snacks instead of a few heavy meals. In more serious cases it may be necessary to resort to surgery to remove the affected area of stomach lining or cut the nerves that trigger off the digestive juices.

HERNIAS

What is a hernia?

A *hernia* occurs when an internal organ becomes displaced and is no longer contained in the correct body cavity. The most common example is when the muscles of the abdomen give way and a loop of the intestine protrudes, but there are many other forms including part of the stomach slipping up past the diaphragm (a mild complaint which often passes unnoticed) and part of the intestine protruding into the upper thigh through the opening for the femoral artery (a complaint mainly found in women). There is a specific type, the *inguinal hernia*, which often affects men. The inguinal canal is the passage down which the testicles descend just before birth and which later houses the spermatic cord and blood vessels. When this type of hernia occurs, part of the intestine protrudes down the canal and into the scrotum.

What causes it?

Congenital hernias can occur when certain muscle structures are weak at birth, but they mostly happen in later life when you begin to lose muscle tone in the natural course of aging. They can also be caused by any form of heavy activity including physical work, lifting weights, strenuous sports, or even violent fits of coughing if the muscles are weak or strained.

What are the symptoms?

These depend on the type of hernia, but there is usually a pain or an ache, pressure in the area and a gurgling feeling in the organ under strain. It can come on gradually, with a slow swelling and worsening symptoms, or it can happen quite suddenly with the feeling that something has "given way." The digestion is often interrupted, with symptoms of constipation.

What is the treatment?

Mild hernias are sometimes held in place with a belt or truss. But so long as it is there, the hernia is in danger of being strangulated, so doctors prefer to repair them surgically by restoring the organ to its proper place and stitching up the opening.

Can a hernia be dangerous?

An organ which has slipped slightly out of place is one thing; it can fairly easily be pushed back. But a strangulated hernia can become acutely inflamed and painful. If it is squeezed tight between muscles, the blood supply to it may be cut off. Without blood, the strangulated part of the hernia rapidly becomes gangrenous. This can cause death within a few days.

THE PROSTATE

What is the prostate?

The *prostate* is a bunch of glands, roughly the size of a chestnut, bound together with muscle tissues and located immediately below the bladder in the lower abdomen. It is wrapped around the top end of the urethra, the tube that takes the urine from the bladder down through the penis. This is why urinary problems are usually the first sign of prostate trouble. The prostate is also adjacent to the wall of the rectum and it can easily be felt by a finger inserted in the anus.

What does it do?

The most obvious function of the prostate is mixing the seminal fluid and producing the mucus-like liquid in which the sperm swim. This fluid is produced continuously, at a normal rate of five to thirty drops an hour and with much larger amounts during sexual excitement. Most of the overflow is discharged a little at a time in the urine. During ejaculation the prostate muscles contract and pump the stored fluid together with the sperm and secretions from the seminal vesicles through small valves into the urethra.

The prostate also makes and releases hormones as part of the elaborate control system of urinary and genital functions.

Doctors now admit that it is one of the most important and least understood of sexual organs, although its anatomy was not adequately worked out until the early 1970s and most of the previous textbooks are very misleading. The medical profession has a lot to answer for in this respect. For instance, although prostate cancer is now replacing cancer of the colon as the second most common form of this disease after lung cancer, only 10 percent of the available anti-cancer drugs had been tested on it up to 1974. But medical research is now catching up, and the introduction of new drugs for bacterial prostitis is a hopeful sign.

What should I do if I have signs of urinary trouble?

If you are worried about possible symptoms, you should consult a doctor. The symptoms may indicate problems such as an inflamed urethra or VD rather than prostate trouble. Even if there is nothing wrong, the worry is worth curing.

But it is as well to bear in mind that there are reasons for some symptoms which are unconnected with any diseases. Changes of weather (or changes of climate if you are on holiday) can effect urinary habits; caffeine in tea and coffee can send you more often to the bathroom; stress and anxiety can have the same effect; and if you are getting on in years, you must ruefully admit that the muscles, even the internal ones, are not what they were.

Does the frequency of sex affect the prostate?

In the past it has been suggested that a possible prostate disorder, *congestive prostatosis*, might be caused by too much or too little sex. The theory is that total abstinence can create a backlog of seminal fluid which causes inflammation – the so-called "priest's disease" – and that overindulgence, usually by masturbating, can overstrain the prostate. This diagnosis is more moralistic than medical and there is little evidence for it. There is even some doubt whether "congestive prostatosis" exists as an identifiable complaint.

The fact is that the prostate continually refreshes its supplies, and discharges the old fluid and infertile sperm during urination. As for overstraining, the prostate is a tough and flexible organ which can stand up to all but the most alarming changes in sexual habits.

What are the signs that something is wrong with the prostate?

Because of its position, any swelling or inflammation of the prostate is likely to affect the flow of urine. So urinary problems are usually the first sign of trouble.

In a mild form these could consist of difficulty in passing urine and a burning sensation when you do manage it, incomplete passing of urine resulting in embarrassing dribbles afterward, and because of the partial retention, the need to go more often, especially at night. In more advanced cases there may be chills and fevers, the passing of blood in the urine and pain in the area of the bladder or the perineal (the area between the scrotum and the anus). If these symptoms are ignored they may develop into a blockage causing the complete retention of urine. This is an excrutiating condition which no one could possibly ignore and is always treated as a medical emergency.

What can go wrong with the prostate?

There are three prostate problems – bacterial infection (*prostatitis*), enlargement (*hypertrophy*) and *cancer*.

Like the lungs and the kidney and other internal organs, the prostate can become infected by bacteria. The symptoms are inflammation, chills and fever, and the bacteria most likely to be responsible are gonorrhea and the colon bacilli e.coli. The e.coli are a harmless and useful part of the digestive system but can cause considerable damage if they get into other parts of the body and are responsible for about 80 percent of acute prostatitis.

This disease can affect one at any age, but the prostate problem normally associated with older people, and which affects nearly half the men over the age of fifty, is *benign prostatic hypertrophy* (BPH). It is probably caused by a hormone imbalance, although there is an outside chance that it is the work of some as yet undiscovered virus. The symptoms resemble prostatitis but without any sign of the bacteria or resulting fever, and in some cases the prostate can swell up to the size of a large grapefuit. However, BPH is usually treated long before it reaches this dramatic stage.

Although it is much less common than infections or BPH, the most widely feared prostate problem is probably cancer. The glandular tissue of the prostate resembles that of a woman's breast and the cancers are similar, but so far there has been no male equivalent to the publicity and mass screening to detect early breast cancer. However, it is as well to remember that cancer differs widely in severity and the speed at which it develops from person to person. Only in the most extreme cases is the surgical removal of the prostate required, and this in turn is not necessarily as drastic as it sounds. The symptoms of cancer are initially the same as BPH, but a doctor would be able to detect the distinctive, hard, irregular lumps during a rectal examination, and this would be followed by detailed clinical tests.

What is the risk of contracting these diseases?

By far the most common is BPH, which affects roughly half of all men over the age of fifty (US statistics). The incidence of prostatitis was declining in the 1950s but has risen sharply in the last fifteen years and the proportion of gonorrhea infections has increased, possibly reflecting the greater sexual freedom in recent years.

The figures for prostate cancer are also rising, with 60,000 new cases reported in the US in 1976, but it still only represents a small percentage of prostate sufferers. Fewer than 5 percent of the 250,000 operations carried out annually in the US for the removal of the prostate were for cancer.

What treatments are available for prostate diseases?

Prostatitis can usually be cured very rapidly with combinations of antibiotics, especially with the use of a new drug called TMP-SMZ, although there is a chronic form of the disease which is more resistant. Surgery is not even considered for prostatitis because of the risk of spreading the infection.

BPH is treated by one of a range of surgical techniques, including cryogenic probes and cauterization, which cut away surplus glandular material. If the prostate is greatly enlarged it may have to be removed.

Cancer, of course, can now call on a whole battery of

modern techniques including surgery, radiation treatment
(both internal and external) and what is probably the most
extraordinary medical treatment in the world – bombardment
by a stream of sub-nuclear particles from a linear accelerator,
such as that recently, and successfully, undergone by a US
Secretary of the Interior.

The Heart
and
Heart Disease

Any short account of heart disease is chilling. It is still the unknown, a plague, confused in many people's minds by the sort of myths and misinformation which once surrounded the Black Death, and which a catalog of medical terms and technology does nothing to dispel.

The almost unbelievable fact that it is the one disease in the world in which the odds are actually on your getting it. It is a disease, not caused by an external, alien source like bacteria, that can be fought and eliminated, but by our own tastes and habits. A short account can only cover the facts. It leaves no room to reassure the anxious about the extraordinary recuperative powers of the human body, or convince the skeptical that it really can happen to them. There is no space for questions such as why almost every government in the western world licenses the sale of poisonous, addictive drugs made by tobacco corporations, brewers and distillers, or how much the vast profits from such industries actually amount to. Nor can we examine the notion that the tastes and habits which are killing us are conditioned by a vast convenience-food industry, with the help of the advertising agencies it hires.

But the most important omission of all is how easy it would be, how reasonable and sane and simple it would be, to change it.

Should I take heart disease seriously? I feel fit and healthy and there seems no reason to worry about it.

The blunt answer is that you should, because you are likely to die from it. In spite of all the advances of medical science this century (including heart transplants) the average life expectancy of a forty-year-old male American is no higher than it was in 1900, and the main reason for this is cardiovascular disease. At present about 20 million people suffer from it, and $1\frac{1}{2}$ million are killed by it, in America each year. The figures may be even higher because upward of a quarter of the US population show high risk symptoms such as obesity or high blood pressure. In 1972, cardiovascular disease was responsible for 53 percent of all deaths in America (compared with 17.5 percent from cancer). In other words, the casualty list of the entire Vietnam war was less than 20 percent of the casualties from heart disease in the USA *in one year*. (National Center for Health Statistics, DHEW US Public Health Dept. 1972.)

What is the heart and what can go wrong with it?

The heart is one of the most efficient machines in existence: a self-repairing, reciprocal pump circulating blood through 60,000 miles of flexible tubes, from arteries an inch in diameter to capillaries so fine that ten of them are no thicker than a hair. It is self-regulating, with a built-in electrical timing device running off a chemical battery and accurate to within 1/50,000th of a second. It can vary its output from five to twelve gallons a minute, directing it to different parts of the system as required, pumping the equivalent of $1\frac{1}{2}$ million gallons a year or, during a lifetime, enough blood to fill the fuel tanks of a fleet of 2,100, four-engined Boeing 747 jets.

The heart system can only do this because it has evolved an immensely complicated system of checks and controls, and some very refined technology such as the super-smooth lining of blood vessels which allows almost frictionless flow. It is controlled by part of the central nervous system, acting as its computer, and also by a system of chemical messengers in the blood itself, both of which provide information feedback on the state of the system and the amount of blood required by each organ.

If anything goes wrong, say the feedback produces inaccurate information or the super-smooth lining (the *endothalium*) gets damaged, there can be a cumulative effect which puts the whole system under strain. This is what happens with heart disease. It may be a fatty deposit on the endothalium, or muscle weakened by infection, or the malfunction of a chemical signal, which starts the trouble, but sooner or later it will affect the two basic conditions on which the whole system operates – sufficient energy for the heart to work, and the accurate regulation of the system. Without sufficient blood supply the heart cannot pump and without proper coordination the pressure and flow cannot be regulated. When any of these things happen, the heart is strained and may be damaged, but it does not fail immediately.

As the disease runs its course, the arteries may continue to clog up, blood pressure rise and the muscles wear out, but the heart continues working. However, it gets progressively less and less effective, and this exacerbates the original trouble. With cause and effect linked in a vicious circle, one part or another of the system eventually fails. The blood supply to some area may be cut off or the heart itself seize up, with catastrophic results.

What are the main forms of heart disease?

There are seven or eight major problems likely to occur in the heart system. The heart may be defective to begin with (*congenital heart disease*), or its muscles weakened by infection (*heart muscle disease* or *myocardiopathy*). The endothalium lining can be damaged in a number of ways by high blood pressure (*hypertension*), the scars left after an infection (*rheumatic heart disease*), or by being blocked by fatty deposits (*arteriosclerosis*). The arteries may also lose their flexibility (*atheroma* or *hardening of the arteries*). Many of the diseases result in (or are the result of) the failure of the control systems to expand and contract blood vessels. When the muscle of the heart itself is deprived of blood in this way it can give rise to severe chest pains (*angina*).

Many of these complaints are interrelated and one can often produce others. Some have specific causes and cures, but the two most common – hypertension and a combination of atheroma and arteriosclerosis called *atherosclerosis* – have complex and often unknown origins. However, they all have the same result in the end, if they are not treated or, better still, avoided.

What is the difference between strokes, heart attacks and coronaries?

These are different forms of systems' failure which result from heart disease. For instance, a blood clot can form at a point where an artery is almost completely blocked or the flow is very slow. This stops the blood supply to any organ or tissue beyond it and is known as *thrombosis* or (if it happens in the artery supplying the heart itself) *coronary thrombosis*. Coronary thrombosis is what is usually meant by a "heart attack." Sometimes a lump of cellullar debris or the remains of an old blood clot will be swept along until it gets stuck in a smaller blood vessel and produces another kind of blockage called an *embolism*. The trouble with an embolus is that though it may start in the extremities, such as a leg, it can move through the body collecting material and getting bigger until it finally clogs an important part of the system like the lungs (*pulmonary embolism*).

When a thrombus or embolus cut off the blood supply to tissue, it dies and is replaced by scar tissue – a process called *infarction*. Not every thrombosis is fatal. In fact it is common for your heart muscle to suffer several minor infarctions before you are forty which you do not even notice. But coronary thrombosis becomes progressively more severe as you get older.

A *stroke* is what happens when the blood supply to your brain is cut off by thrombosis or, more rarely, when a blood vessel ruptures and hemorrhages in the skull. The death of brain tissue obviously has profound effects on the whole body and stroke victims are often paralyzed or deprived of other faculties such as speech.

Thrombosis can happen very suddenly, but *heart failure* usually signals its presence in advance. It occurs when the heart cannot keep pace with the demands made on it by heart disease, high blood pressure or extreme physical exertion, and the pumping muscle, weakened or damaged by in-farctions, finally seizes up.

If for any of these reasons the heart stops beating there are two to three minutes before irreversible damage sets in and, if it is not restarted within four minutes, you die.

What are the symptoms of thrombosis or heart attacks?

The classic symptoms are pains in the chest and shortness of breath, accompanied by dizziness, prolonged fatigue and irregular heartbeats; but these are so vague that they could easily be misunderstood. It is essential to get medical advice if you are in doubt because only a physician can assess the other risk factors, take your blood pressure and make diagnostic tests. The nature and sequence of the pains, for instance, is all important. You might be alarmed by sharp stabbing pains in the area of the heart, accompanied by what feel like palpitations, but they are likely to be no more than air trapped in the stomach or the colon pressing up against the diaphragm. On the other hand, a sense of pressure or burning behind the breast bone, particularly on the left hand side, could be angina. A pain in the chest can also be caused by indigestion. Yet the feeling of indigestion can actually be the sign of an impending heart attack – if it is different from what you are used to or changes its character within half an hour from a stomach pain to heaviness in the chest radiating to your neck. There again, an unexpected attack of heartburn, followed by several days of paleness and lassitude, could be a warning to expect a second episode leading to a heart attack.

Because it is so difficult to diagnose heart trouble, if you are in pain it is much better to let your physician decide how serious it is.

How can you tell if someone is suffering an attack?

In the case of heart failure there is breathlessness and chest pains. One side of the heart usually fails first and the pressure builds up as the other continues to function. The rhythm of the heartbeat is slow, or very fast, or irregular. The legs and ankles tend to swell up and the lungs to fill with fluid.

Heart attacks tend to happen abruptly and are accompanied by breathlessness, dizziness, cold sweat and severe pain. If it is a stroke, the patient may be unable to move or speak.

Are there any "early warning" signs of heart disease?

The problem with many heart diseases, such as atherosclerosis, is that they creep up on you unawares, developing for many years before physical signs are noticeable. So your doctor will be as interested in your past history as your present symptoms. The only way to identify this sort of heart disease in advance is to calculate, from known risk factors, how likely you are to get it.

Genetic abnormalities can usually be identified by clinical tests and certain diseases such as rheumatic fever are known to be likely causes of heart trouble later.

What are the main "risk factors" of heart disease?

Risk factors are warning signs which can double, triple – or multiply up to twenty times – the chances of having heart disease. They include high blood pressure, increased levels of cholesterol in the blood, your age (especially if you are over forty), your sex (if you are male), smoking, drinking, over-eating or eating the wrong diet, lack of exercise and a stressful lifestyle.

What is cholesterol?

Cholesterol is an important chemical which the body needs as the base from which to make hormones and bile salts for the digestive process. Some of it comes from our food and some is produced by the liver, and there is a more or less constant, and necessary, amount circulating through the bloodstream to various destinations. Along the way some of it filters through the walls of the arteries into the lymph system. This filtration process works well under normal circumstances, but if there is too much cholesterol or the blood pressure tries to force too much material through the filter, it will eventually clog up and cells will be deposited on the walls of the artery.

Since the pressure on the filtering system can start a deposit, the fatty streaks usually occur first where the arteries divide or have a sharp curve. Like a river, these are the points where the current is strongest. Another point where the pressure is high and deposits likely to occur is in the main arteries, especially the coronary artery itself, which will pump blood several feet into the air if it is severed.

Is it sensible to have regular medical check-ups?

It depends on your state of health and how many risk factors apply to you. If you are in a dangerous age bracket and social background, smoke, drink and are overweight, you should have check-ups at least every six months, and watch for symptoms. No one will accuse you of hypochondria and it may save your life.

What is the "heart rate"?

When you are relaxed your heart beats sixty to seventy times a minute, pushing out about three to four ounces of blood each time. Under physical stress such as running, this rises to 180 or 190 beats a minute, by which time the heart is pumping forty pints a minute. The arteries expand as each surge passes through, and this can be felt as the pulse.

If you want to take your own pulse, position your hand palm upward, and feel the side of your wrist away from the body. Only feel with your fingertips because the artery runs up into the thumb and the two beats could be confused.

What is blood pressure?

When a doctor checks your blood pressure he takes two measurements – the high pressure in the system when the heart contracts (*systole*) and the minimum pressure (*diastole*) when it relaxes. The first varies from 100 to 120 Hg and the lower, diastolic pressure is normally 70 to 80 Hg. A physician writes this as, say, 100/70 or 120/80, and what he is looking at are not the figures themselves but the difference between them. In good health the average or mean between the figures stays the same, regardless of an increased flow. When the proportion varies, it is a sign of trouble. If the diastolic pressure is too low it is a sign that the blood flow to the heart might be impaired. If it is too high it indicates an increased resistance to flow throughout the body which could be straining the heart. Chronically high blood pressure, with permanently increased resistance to flow, is called *hypertension*.

Are men more likely to suffer from heart disease than women?

The cardiovascular system is much the same in men and women, although on average a woman's heart is one fifth smaller and produces six to eight more beats a minute. But there is a marked difference between them when it comes to heart disease. Whether it is due to differences in their metabolism or lifestyles, fewer women experience coronary heart complaints, and do so much later in life, than men. From the age of fifteen to twenty-five you are 50 percent more likely to suffer heart disease than a woman, but for most of your life, from twenty-five to sixty-five years of age, you are more than two or three times as susceptible to it.

Beyond the age of sixty-five the figures level out but it is only in the seventies that women are more at risk.

What is the reason for this difference?

At first it was assumed that it must reflect some difference in their metabolism, and there is certainly some evidence which links the phenomenon to specific male and female chemistry. For instance, women who have had their ovaries removed before menopause are as much at risk as men in comparable age groups. This seemed to be confirmed by a classic series of experiments carried out during the 1950s by Dr. Louis Katz of the Michael Reese Research Institute of Chicago. He showed that arteriosclerosis in chicks, caused by a high-cholesterol diet, could be prevented by giving them the female hormone, estrogen. The natural conclusion would be that women are somehow "protected" from heart disease by their hormones until they reach menopause. But this cannot be the only cause or there would be a more abrupt change in the statistics at that age. Women are certainly more susceptible to heart disease after menopause, but the figures change gradually as they get older.

The hormone theory received a severe setback when subsequent experiments using estrogen on men showed no signs of reducing their rate of heart disease. These tests were suspended altogether in 1975, when a large-scale experiment in the USA revealed that men treated with estrogen after surviving one heart attack were more likely to have a second and had a *higher* mortality rate. (Coronary Drug Project. Study of 8,000 survivors of heart attacks sponsored by the US National Heart and Lung Institute, 1975.)

This discrepancy between the sexes is probably the result of a number of factors, including body chemistry and genetic mechanisms (women can be the carrier of hereditary diseases like hemophilia without being affected by them) coupled with the fact that they are less likely to be exposed to certain risk factors.

Differences in their lifestyles may be a key factor, because curiously enough there is a change in recent figures, showing that the differential is narrowing and more women are now getting heart disease. This could reflect the fact that more women smoke and drink, and tend to compete more with men for high-stress competitive jobs. But if the risk factors are now beginning to outweigh women's natural immunity, it would be an ironic price to pay for their liberation.

What is an electrocardiograph?

An *electrocardiograph* is a device for measuring the electrical impulses of the heart muscle, which enables a physician to determine the presence, extent and location of muscle damage, analyze irregular heart beats and diagnose cases of heart attack. Sensors are attached to the chest, ankles and wrists of the patient and the signals fed into a machine which records the fluctuations of electrical potential as a series of wavy lines on a long strip of paper (an *electrocardiogram* or EKG).

Although the electrocardiograph is a useful monitoring device to be found in most doctors' surgeries, it is not a crystal ball. An EKG does not record the conditions of the coronary arteries or the extent of arteriosclerosis which may have caused the heart attack, and cannot be used to predict the next one.

Is there any means of detecting blockages in arteries?

Yes, the commonly used method is an X-ray technique called *angiography* or *coronary arteriography*, which requires a dye that is opaque to X-rays to be fed into the bloodstream so that it outlines the shape of the internal walls of the artery. The dye cannot be injected into the whole system because the resulting X-rays would be too confusing. So in order to isolate one blood vessel out of thousands, the dye is fed through a tube to a point just above the suspected blockage before it is released. To reach the coronary artery, which is the usual target, the tube, or *catheter*, is inserted into a blood vessel in the arm or groin and then gently pushed through the system to a point above the aorta.

The dye is harmless and the operation, however horrifying it sounds, is painless. But it is a complicated procedure and is normally only used when surgery is being considered and the doctors want to see what they are up against.

Where does the blood go, and how long does it take to circulate?

The ten pints of blood you have in your body are constantly being redistributed to various parts. For instance, more goes to your stomach while you are digesting a meal or to your legs when you are running. But on average, when you are at rest and between meals, the brain gets 15 percent, the muscles 15 percent, the intestines 30 percent, the kidneys 20 percent, the skin and skeleton 10 percent and the heart itself 5 percent. If all the blood vessels dilated at once it would require 90 pints a minute to fill the system, but since the heart's maximum capacity is about 50 pints a minute, the pressure would drop to zero and the individual would bleed to death into his own blood vessels.

The longest journey the blood does, from heart to toe and back again, takes about sixteen seconds at rest. The return journey to the brain takes about eight seconds, and the short trip to the lungs only takes about six seconds.

What is angina?

Angina is a severe pain in the chest which results from a lack of blood supply to the heart muscle. When an organ needs more blood, the flow is increased by an intricate signaling system of nerves and chemicals, called *autoregulation*, which rapidly dilates or contracts the smaller blood vessels. If the system fails or the blood vessels are not elastic enough to expand, the organ is starved of oxygen. When this happens to the heart itself, the muscles fail to contract (and can even bulge in the opposite direction) and the nerve endings become irritated, producing a feeling of "heaviness" and pain in the chest called *angina pectoris* (angina is a word used to describe any pain produced by a muscular spasm).

Angina is not a disease so much as a symptom, like cramp, which results when the system is under strain for some other reason. It usually occurs after additional exertion such as physical exercise, or even a large meal. In severe cases it can occur when you are at rest.

Is it possible to have angina for a long time without it getting worse?

If you suffer from a chronic heart disease, you may also suffer from angina for years. Under proper medication some heart complaints can be contained and their effects reduced by a careful diet and lifestyle. But most of them are progressive, so that the disease, and the angina which accompanies it, is likely to get steadily worse.

What is hypertension?

Hypertension is a condition of permanent or semi-permanent high blood pressure, which puts a strain on the heart and promotes atherosclerosis by wear and tear on the blood vessels. In the early stages, the blood pressure may only rise during periods of physical activity, but later it occurs even when you are resting (*stable hypertension*). It is not necessarily linked to the aging process and often starts in your thirties, although it can occur at any age.

Hypertension results from a failure of one or another of the control and feedback mechanisms which balance the blood supply. These work by constricting or dilating the blood vessels, adjusting the caliber by nerve impulses from the central nervous system and chemical messengers released into the bloodstream by various glands, the kidneys and the heart itself. The two mechanisms provide a back-up to each other, monitoring the pressure through the nervous system and kidneys. This takes care of temporary fluctuations, but there is also a system controlling long-term changes, from day to night, or over the seasons, by regulating the amount of water in the blood and tissues (*blood volume*).

It is essential that all these delicate interracting mechanisms remain in balance. If something goes wrong, for any of a score of reasons, anywhere in the system, hypertension can result.

What are the causes of hypertension?

In some cases it is possible to identify a breakdown in the chain of communication, but most of the time, in about 85 percent of cases of hypertension, the system gradually goes wrong, like a clock gaining on itself, and the pressure rises without any obvious symptoms.

One of the few specific causes so far discovered is related to the kidney. If there is arteriosclerosis blocking its blood supply upstream, the kidney registers an artificially low blood pressure. It then tries to remedy matters by releasing a flood of chemical messengers (*renin*) to increase the pressure of its own blood supply and creates unnecessarily high blood pressure elsewhere. Pressure on the adrenal gland, such as could be caused by a tumor, has the same effect, releasing another chemical signal (*aldosterone*) involved in pressure regulation. The nervous system tries to correct the results, but the adrenal gland and the kidney, still receiving misinformation, continue to put out a barrage of blood-borne messengers which overide the other signals, and the hypertension is increased.

What are the risk factors for hypertension?
Are there any "early warning" signs?

Hypertension can have such complex causes that, like

coronary heart disease, they can only be approached by statistical evidence showing who is most likely to get it.

Heredity seems to play a moderately important role. Experiments on identical twins indicate that there may be a genetic predisposition to high blood pressure, but it is difficult to separate this from possible causes in the lifestyle or environment shared by the same family. The black population in the US has higher blood pressure, on average, than whites, which would appear to be a racial characteristic. But the black population in "underdeveloped" countries in Africa show markedly less hypertension than the population of most western countries, which seems to throw the blame back on our "civilized" living standards.

Various lifestyle factors which might put you at risk have been suggested: overeating, for instance (overweight people have a higher rate of hypertension), or soft drinking water (the chemicals it dissolves from lead pipes have been shown to cause kidney damage and high blood pressure in rats), or too much salt in your diet (fishing communities and others who eat excessively salty food display a very high rate of blood pressure) – and there may be many others.

The salt factor may be a symptom as well as a cause. The retention of extra water and salt in body tissues is an early sign of hypertension, and by increasing the total blood volume it stimulates the heart to work harder, thereby pushing up the pressure.

Is there a cure for hypertension?

Medication has proved very effective in controlling hypertension. Although little is known about what triggers it off, quite a lot is known about how the mechanism is maintained. Once high blood pressure has been identified, the chain reaction of cause and effect throughout the system can be halted by the use of drugs to modify and correct the internal signals. This will not cure it, but it reduces the risk of other heart complaints developing and makes life tolerable for the sufferer.

More than 25 million Americans suffer from some form of hypertension and the problem is so enormous that some governments are considering major health programs to combat it. One of the largest ever clinical trials was launched in the United Kingdom in 1978, to study the effects of a drug called propanolol (which dilates blood vessels and reduces blood pressure) on a group of 36,000 volunteers suffering from mild hypertension. But prevention, as always, is better than cure.

What is congenital heart disease?

Congenital heart disease is when the heart fails to develop properly before birth. It covers phenomena such as "hole-in-the-heart babies" and affects about 70,000 children born each year in the USA. Sometimes the heart condition is only part of an overall genetic abnormality involving the central nervous system and inherited from the mother's genes. But more often it is the result of damage done to the fetus in the womb. This will occur if the mother suffers from diabetes or hypertension, or contracts certain virus infections such as scarlet fever, during pregnancy. In rarer cases the same effects can be produced by taking certain drugs.

In some instances congenital heart diseases can be corrected by surgery. Modern techniques are so sophisticated that surgeons can virtually rebuild a patient's heart. But congenital diseases are likely to have so many tragic and incurable side effects that prevention is the only answer. The incidence of these abnormalities would be drastically reduced if parents underwent genetic tests and counselling before marriage and pregnant mothers were fully informed and properly protected.

Are other heart diseases inheritable? Can there be a predisposition to heart disease which runs in families?

A popular misconception about heart disease is that heredity is all-important. It is commonly believed that if your parents and grandparents suffered from it, then so will you. But this is only partly true and is often no more than a fatalistic excuse to do nothing about it. The influence of heredity on congenital heart disease and hypertension has already been mentioned. But they are only part of the problem and are usually linked to other factors. In most other cases heart disease is not inevitable, and frequently avoidable. There may be a family tendency to be overweight, but this can be either improved by a sensible diet or made much worse by bad eating habits. Your metabolism may be liable to increase cholesterol levels, but until this is related to age, sex and other risk factors, there is no way of knowing whether it will produce arteriosclerosis. The habits that you develop as a child can be more dangerous than any biological inheritance.

What is heart muscle disease?

Heart muscle disease is a relatively rare disease which inflames and weakens the muscle which does the pumping. The causes are largely unknown, although it is thought that some kind of virus infection may be responsible. It is a progressive disease. As the heart muscle gets weaker, it impairs the blood supply to other organs and can result in acute or chronic heart failure.

Among the risk factors associated with the disease, the most serious is alcoholism. It is the main cause in some cases, but even a small intake of alcohol can exacerbate an existing condition.

Does alcohol affect all heart diseases? Should I give up even light occasional drinking?

Steady drinking, even of small amounts, affects the central nervous system, heart, liver, brain and kidneys. As little as a 2-ounce shot of whiskey will temporarily decrease the efficiency of the heart muscle.

But the cumulative effect is more important than occasional binges. Alcoholic heart muscle disease (*myocardiopathy*) is more common among social drinkers who can take several drinks "without noticing any effect," than the people who seldom drink, and tend to overdo it when they do.

Alcohol is also an important risk factor in atherosclerosis, where a drink before a meal can increase the cholesterol intake from the food, especially if it contains meat.

What is rheumatic heart disease?

Rheumatic heart disease affects about 1 percent of the US population and is the main cause of heart trouble in children. It results from rheumatic fever, which can affect the heart as well as inflaming the joints. The heart can fail as a direct result of the disease, but more often it leaves the tissues scarred and thickened and liable to heart failure later in life.

Another widespread form is caused by a bacterial throat infection (*hemolytic streptococcus*). "Strep throat," as it is sometimes called, is not directly responsible, but it leaves bacterial toxins circulating in the blood which inflame the lining of the arteries, particularly around the heart valves. When the inflammation dies down, it leaves scars and loss of elasticity.

What causes arteries to harden, and why is it dangerous?

Age is one factor. Like all tissues, arteries tend to lose their muscular tone with age. Rather like an old rubber hose, they become stiffer and less flexible as we grow older. But this is seldom the only cause of arteriosclerosis. Any kind of damage, such as the inflammation caused by certain infectious diseases or a tear in the lining, will leave behind scar tissue that has no elasticity and cannot respond to variations in the blood flow. When additional oxygen is required in that part of the body, the hardened arteries cannot expand to let the extra blood through, and the pressure inevitably builds up.

The most common reason for hardened arteries is the accumulation of material on their walls. These are not only inflexible in themselves, but stiffen the walls with deposits of calcium and reduce the diameter of the tube so that even if the artery manages to expand, the blood still cannot get through.

What is the deposit that clogs the arteries?

Apart from traces of salts and other chemicals, the deposit looks like a yellow mushy foam of cellular material containing fat particles and cholesterol. The first layer is trapped in the tissues of the artery wall and produces a thin, barely visible deposit called a fatty streak. As the build-up proceeds, the endothalium lining attempts to cover it. But when it becomes too thick and bumpy the lining will eventually tear or crack, producing ideal conditions for a blood clot to develop.

At what age are you most likely to develop atherosclerosis?

If you develop heart disease in later life, the first symptoms can occur unnoticed when you are comparatively young. The post-mortems on young soldiers who died in the Korean War showed that 77 percent of them had fatty streaks and early signs of atherosclerosis, and 15 percent had at least one serious blockage in an artery.

If atherosclerosis can develop without your knowing it, when do the symptoms first appear?

The coronary system has a large reserve capacity and chest pains are not usually felt until the inner caliber, or bore, of the arteries has been reduced by 50 percent. By this time you can assume that the system is badly damaged, and likely to get worse. When the obstruction reduces the flow by about 70 percent, the situation becomes critical and major symptoms such as blood clotting may occur.

What are the symptoms of atherosclerosis?

If an artery is obstructed, the part of your body it supplies will feel the effects long before it is eventually cut off. These effects are sometimes thought of as associated diseases. For instance, if the leg muscles are affected it can produce a severe pain in the calf, or the whole leg, while walking, which disappears after a few minutes' rest. If the obstruction is bad enough it can hurt even when resting and the skin may be pale and cold.

If the obstruction is reducing the blood supply to the brain, it can impair other functions and cause slurred speech and temporary disorientation.

The other symptoms a physician would look for are incidents of angina, a history of previous heart attacks and abnormal EKG readings.

What are the causes, or risk factors, of atherosclerosis?

There is no single cause of atherosclerosis and the exact mechanisms which trigger off the disease are not yet fully understood. But, like hypertension, there are risk factors which not so much add up as multiply together to make it more likely that you will get the disease.

You may have a metabolic problem, such as diabetes or certain kidney diseases, which could increase the cholesterol levels in your blood; you may have inherited a tendency to make smaller fat and cholesterol molecules (*low density lipoproteins*) which are more likely to be deposited in the arterial wall; your diet may be high in cholesterol, which increases the level in your system; or you may lead a sedentary life and not take the sort of exercise which burns up fats and flexes the heart system. Both drinking and smoking are now thought to be major risk factors, and if these factors are combined with a pattern of psychological stress and high blood pressure, you are many times more likely to suffer from atherosclerosis than anyone else of your age and sex.

Is there a cure for atherosclerosis?

There are no drugs which will remove the deposits of atherosclerosis or soften up hardened arteries, although there have been cases where a combination of carefully controlled diet and drugs to reduce the level of cholesterol in the blood has resulted in the deposits gradually reducing of their own accord. There are also drugs (called *anti-coagulants*) which thin down the blood to stop it clotting and therefore avoid the worst effects of atherosclerosis. But these are palliative measures which are simply intended to slow down or stop the spread of the disease. Once the deposits have been laid down they are usually there to stay.

When the arteries are so badly scarred or blocked that there is a threat of thrombosis, the only option is surgery.

What about surgery? Can the deposits be cut away?

Before describing the surgical treatments which are available, it is worth mentioning the automatic treatment which every-one has for free – the heart's extraordinary ability to repair itself. If an artery is blocked, and the blood can find no alternative route, the artery can actually grow a new connection to another artery and bypass the blockage (*collateral circulation*). How it does this, or knows where the connection should go, is still a mystery, but it is definitely a last resort and only occurs when the heart muscle has been repeatedly starved of oxygen. Perhaps even more surprisingly, there is some evidence that a rough hard-working life involving a lot of manual labor can prevent heart disease in some social groups, by developing collateral circulation before it is needed.

There is a surgical operation sometimes used to remove arterial deposits (*coronary endarterectomy*). It consists of injecting carbon dioxide gas into the walls of the artery to loosen deposits, cutting them free inside and pulling them out through a small slit. However, the operation is rarely performed because the problem is seldom caused by a single obstruction. Most of the surgical procedures attempt to copy nature by building in new blood vessels. Sometimes a comparatively unimportant artery under the breast bone (the *internal mammary artery*) is disconnected at one end and fed into the heart instead. This is called the *Vineberg procedure* and is very effective because the heart apparently accepts this extra supply without difficulty and it eases the pressure on the blocked artery. But the most widely used operation is to graft on a bypass around the damaged section, using natural arteries or veins from the patient's leg, or one of the new artificial arteries made of woven plastic which can be bought by length off the shelf and in a variety of sizes.

How does my diet affect my chances of getting heart disease?

If one had to specify the single most dangerous cause of heart disease, it would probably be a rushed city lunch where social or business drinks are followed by an 8-oz T-bone with French fries and half a lettuce leaf, fruit pie with ice cream, coffee and cream, with cigarettes being smoked before, during and after the meal. Every one of these ingredients is a killer, particularly when repeated day after day, but the point is not just that it is the wrong food, but that there is *too much*. Over-eating is a widespread cause of ill health in most western countries and if it were reduced it would have a marked affect on the statistics for heart disease. Health surveys carried out in Europe during and after World War II showed that the population, and particularly the children, was much healthier in war-time conditions when food was scarce and strictly rationed, than it was in times of peace and plenty. Ironically, the lowest figures for heart disease today come from Third World countries where the people live on the borderline of malnutrition. It is one illness where the villain is not a germ or virus breeding in squalor, but the product of a civilized, ultra-hygienic, consumer society.

But overindulgence is not the only factor; the other half of the heart disease formula is that we eat too much of *the wrong things*. It is not dietary deficiency which causes the disease, but a constant intake of fats which we do not need and cannot digest. That is why a perfectly normal, and otherwise un-exceptional, city lunch can be so dangerous. The T-bone steak was full of saturated fats which hold cholesterol. So were the potatoes if they were fried in animal fat, so was the pie filling, and the pastry, and the ice cream, and the cream in the coffee. And both the alcohol in the drinks and the nicotine in the cigarettes made it easier for them to be added to the blood-stream. There was probably white sugar in the coffee and a white bread roll on a side plate (refined carbohydrates and sugars lack many essential trace minerals), the butter for the roll (all that cholesterol), not to mention the coffee itself (caffeine can produce anxiety, heart palpitations and symptoms of hyperactivity). If there had been a fried egg with the steak, that could have been added to the list because egg yolks are also high in cholesterol.

What is the difference between saturated and polyunsaturated fats?

The two kinds of fat differ in the shape of their molecules. The basic form of both types is a glycerine molecule, with a number of fatty acid molecules attached to it. These in turn have a number of points to which other molecules (such as iodine) can be joined. In the case of *polyunsaturated fats*, these spare connections are available; with *saturated fats*, they are already taken up by hydrogen atoms and this makes them more difficult for our metabolism to break down and absorb. Saturated fats come mainly from meat, animal fat and dairy products, and contain high levels of cholesterol; polyunsaturated fats come mainly from vegetable oils, and some fish oils. Margerine is unsaturated and will not do you any harm; butter is saturated, and will.

I find diets complicated and difficult to follow. Are there any simple, or essential, changes I should make to what I eat?

If you want to lessen your chances of heart disease it is worth the effort. There are many books and leaflets available if you seriously want to do something about it. Unfortunately there is not space here to give the full details or suggest menus, but if you want a rule of thumb guide, these are the points to look out for.

Don't overeat. It may sound complicated, but it is worth while getting to know the calorie system and having some idea of what you are eating. Apart from improving your health, it actually saves money to eat less.

Try to avoid cholesterol heavy foods. There is no need to be obsessive about it and cut them out altogether. Just cut down. Dairy products, eggs and meat are the worst offenders (even lean meat contains 15 percent saturated fats). Stick to chicken, fish and just three eggs a week, if you can manage it. And if you must fry them, use vegetable oil. Go easy on dairy products, such as unskimmed milk and butter

Use brown sugar and bread.

Eat all the fruit and vegetables you can. Not because they are an antidote to heart disease, but because they are harmless, healthy and taste good.

Can the lack of certain vitamins affect heart disease?

A balanced vitamin intake is certainly essential for your general good health and vitamins are simple to understand compared with the more complicated diet-math. But they can be misleading taken in isolation. And, once again, we tend to suffer from overdoses rather than deficiency. They have almost achieved the status of a cult these days and have been seized on by the commercial drug industry to market vast quantities of unnecessary products. Among the claims they make is that by taking vitamin C and E tablets you can improve your chances against heart disease, especially atherosclerosis. It would be wonderful if heart disease could be cured with a pill, but unfortunately it cannot. Vitamin C can actually be harmful in large amounts and although our metabolism needs Vitamin E, careful tests have shown no connection with the incidence of heart disease. Regularly taking unprescribed vitamin pills is just another way of filling your body with unwanted chemicals.

I've heard that physical exercise is very important. How does it affect the risk of heart disease?

It is important to remember that exercise is a prevention rather than a cure. If you already have some form of heart disease, it can be dangerous to overexert yourself. It can strain the heart or cause angina, and the amount of exercise you do should be prescribed by your physician.

Except for these special cases, reasonably hard, regular physical exercise is one of the best ways to avoid heart disease. Recent research among longshoremen in San Francisco showed that those with heavier jobs were much less likely to get it than those on lighter work. And similar studies in the southern USA showed that sharecroppers working on the land were less liable to heart complaints than their relatives leading sedentary lives in the towns.

Exercise directly improves the heart and circulatory system in several ways. To start with it strengthens the heart muscle. It also increases the oxygen-carrying capacity of the blood and makes it less likely to coagulate into a clot. By pushing a large amount of blood through the system, the arteries are enlarged and collateral circulation is encouraged to develop. At the same time it loosens up the muscles and flexes the arteries so that they are more elastic, while the increased flow tends to remove cholesterol deposits. All this makes high blood pressure and atherosclerosis less likely to develop.

But it is important to do the right sort of exercise. For instance, exercises which rhythmically tense and relax your muscles (*isotonic exercises*) are more beneficial than those which tense the muscles only to increase their strength (*isometric exercises*) like weight lifting.

Exercise is more valuable if it gets additional oxygen to your muscles for an extended period. A hundred-yard sprint does this, but for such a short period as to be virtually useless. On the other hand, a brisk thirty-minute walk each day will measurably increase your physical fitness.

Perhaps the most important value of exercise is that it burns up fats and calories and helps to reduce your weight. Without it there tends to be a vicious circle where lack of exercise increases your weight, and the more overweight you are, the less exercise you take. Not only will a moderate increase in physical activity reduce your weight (on average it is possible to lose twenty-five pounds in just over four months by ten minutes of jogging a day), but it can actually reduce your calorie intake by suppressing your appetite.

Is it true that business executives and other people in high-pressure jobs are more likely to have heart trouble? How important is psychological stress?

Stress is known to be an important factor in other ailments such as stomach ulcers and there is a widely accepted theory that people with a certain psychological profile in stress positions are more susceptible to heart disease. This group is known as *Type A* and is described as aggressive, impatient and overambitious. More placid and easy-going people are classified as *Type B*. Some specialists believe that Type A behavior is a risk factor in itself and support their views with extensive research showing that there are more Type A people among the victims of heart disease than there are Type B people.

But their conclusion has been challenged, and it has been pointed out that there may be other explanations for the figures. For instance, there may be risk factors in the environment which Type A people tend to inhabit. Ambitious go-getters tend to have executive-style jobs and these are more likely to include excessive social drinking to balance the stress. Or it may be that quiet Type B people develop Type A behavior because they are in competitive jobs. This sort of psycho-dynamic analysis is inevitably rather ambiguous and difficult to check, but so far there is no *specific* evidence to show that Type A people are more at risk. In fact, what evidence there is tends to point the other way. For instance, it definitely is not an "executive's disease." The figures show that people from all classes are equally likely to suffer from it – but then who is to say that the stress of being rich is any worse than the stress of being poor?

What happens after a heart attack or stroke? How long does it take to recover and what sort of limitations does it put on your life?

It depends on how bad the damage was. With a mild attack, you can resume your life a few days or even hours later. Or it may take a slow climb back to normality over many months. It may mean that a wheelchair or a bed has to become your home – but even that represents the singular privilege of still being alive.

But assuming that you have survived – and most heart failures and thromboses are mild enough to give you a second chance – you will be put under strict medical supervision. If you have any sense you will obey it to the letter. The first thing the doctor will say to you is that after a short spell of bed rest, you are to be up and moving about as soon as possible. He will then tell you, especially if you are a Type A personality, that you must learn to relax, whatever it costs you in counting slowly up to ten or giving up weight lifting for golf. It can be difficult to do this consciously, to actually make yourself calm, but there are techniques of auto-suggestion and "concentrative relaxation" which help. You may even find yourself being forcibly taken on a recuperative holiday by well-meaning relatives.

The next thing he will say is that you are to give up smoking, immediately and without argument, and to reduce your drinking habits to a tolerable minimum. He may add that you have to lose weight and go on a "life saver" cholesterol-free diet, and suggest some gentle program of exercises (yoga and tai chi are ideal). He will not tell you to give up sex or sport (provided that neither is too violent) and he will positively urge you not to give up your job (unless it is to change to a less strenuous one). It is important that you don't give up. The anxiety and depression which follow it can do more damage than the original heart attack.

From that point on it is up to you. With a little determination, self-confidence and you should be able to overcome your disabilities. People with strokes have even regained their speech and other faculties by "retraining" unused parts of their brain to take over from damaged areas. If you are lucky you will probably find that all you have lost is a certain elasticity. Your body, with all its complex interlocking systems, is now working on narrower tolerances and is no longer flexible enough to deal with swings and excesses. But provided you keep that delicate balance, there is no reason why you should not lead a happy, productive and extended life.

If you get to like golf, there is no reason why you should not still be walking the links twenty or thirty years later.

When are pacemakers and artificial valves used?
And what about heart transplants? Is there such a thing
as an artificial heart?

Technological miracles tend to become commonplace. Open-heart surgery has come a long way since 1967, when the first human heart was transplanted from the body of a twenty-five-year-old black woman killed in an auto-crash to that of a fifty-three-year-old South African grocer. The heart-lung machine and the new science of "tissue-typing" which made the pioneer work of Dr. Christiaan Barnard (whose middle-aged patient survived eighteen days before dying of pneu-monia) and Dr. Michael DeBakey possible, is now routine, and the heart can be patched up, repaired, rebuilt or replaced more or less as needed. But the operations are expensive and facilities for carrying them out are limited, so they are usually reserved for patients whose hearts are severely damaged, usually by heart attacks.

There are four or five standard repair jobs commonly carried out. If the electrical timing device in the sinus node is damaged, the heart may be beating irregularly (*arrhythmia*). This can be corrected by fitting a pacemaker, which generates similar electrical impulses from an outside supply or special long-life batteries implanted under the skin of the groin or armpit. Another frequent result of heart attacks is damaged tissues. These can result in heavy scars dragging the other muscles out of shape, or a weakened area that balloons out of shape under pressure (an *aneurysm*), or the internal valves may be damaged and not pumping properly. All these can now be repaired by surgery. Artificial valves, working on the same principle as ball-valves on snorkels, can be fitted and ruptured internal partitions patched with woven dacron fabric.

There will certainly be an artificial heart available one day, but for the moment when the heart is damaged beyond repair there is no alternative but the heart transplant operation. The risks are still enormous, but the odds are shortening. The surgery itself is simple and the outstanding problem, that of the "immune reaction" which prevents grafts taking, is now one of the main fields of medical research.

It is odd to think that the heart, which was once considered the most mysterious and complex of organs, should be one of the first and easiest to replace. After all, no one has any idea yet of how to replace the lung or liver tissues (let alone brain cells) with plastic replicas.

Is smoking a risk factor in heart disease?

In addition to its other effects, there is no question that smoking is one of the major risk factors in heart disease. Dr. Alton Ochsner of Tulane Medical School once said, "Smoking may have one virtue. By smoking heavily a man may have a heart attack, but at least he won't live long enough to develop cancer." Since the US Surgeon General's report in 1964, which first put the health warning on cigarette packs, evidence of the connection between smoking and heart disease has been accumulating.

It is known that coronary heart disease occurs, on average, up to seven years earlier in smokers than non-smokers. A single cigarette can bring on an attack of angina and, especially when the heart is already weakened, it increases the chance of heart attacks. Smoking is also directly linked to arteriosclerosis. A recent five-year study by the Mayo Clinic showed that giving up smoking had a marked effect on the course of the disease. Smoking raises the level of cholesterol in the blood, increases the heart rate and promotes high blood pressure.

Unfortunately there is no avoiding the fact. Smoking aggravates almost all cardiovascular conditions and, in some cases, can be the critical factor in a patient's survival.

How does smoking affect the heart system?
What is the connection?

Nicotine is a vasoconstrictive drug which shrinks the smaller blood vessels and increases the blood pressure. Since a single cigarette is known to increase the heart rate for about a quarter of an hour, it was first thought that this strain, constantly repeated throughout the day, might damage the heart system. But the effect is too slight to be a significant factor.

Nicotine is also known to decrease the liver's ability to clear blood fats after a meal, and there may be a link in this respect. But a more likely connection is not the nicotine, but the carbon monoxide you inhale from a cigarette at the same time. The carbon monoxide molecule has an affinity for hemoglobin 250 times stronger than that of oxygen, so that in the lungs it is much more likely to be absorbed into the blood. Because of this, heavy smokers can have as much as 10 percent to 15 percent of their red blood cells bound by carbon monoxide and prevented from doing their job. This could create an oxygen shortage, which in turn would raise the heart rate and blood pressure.

The carbon monoxide factor is doubly dangerous because it sets up a chain reaction in the system. The body will register the oxygen shortage as a lack of red blood cells, and will produce more to make up for this apparent loss. But this would only thicken the blood and make clotting more likely, while the increased viscosity would put further strain on the heart to keep it moving.

The other toxic substances in cigarette smoke, such as carcinogenic tars, produce lung cancer, respiratory diseases and other side effects, and sooner or later these take their toll on the heart system. But it seems as if a combination of nicotine and carbon monoxide do the real and immediate damage.

Drugs

The use of drugs for social and medical purposes is now ubiquitous. In most western countries we live in a drug culture conditioned to a massive intake of hypnotics, alcohol, antibiotics, vitamins, analgesics, nicotine, sedatives, caffeine and hallucinogens. The hard-core fringe of heroin addiction is nothing compared to the saturation-bombing of uppers, downers, slimmers, sleepers, tranquilizers and stimulants consumed in millions, by millions, every day. Drugs to hallucinate, decongest, ovulate, stop ovulating, concentrate, sun-tan and forget, the pill boom goes roaring on unchecked, with new mood-altering miracles rushed to the counters as they are invented.

Almost every society has taken drugs in one form or another, usually intoxicants, but their consumption was always regulated by social forms and traditions. But there has been such an increase in the range and availability of new drugs that all the traditional controls are breaking down. Illegal drugs cannot be licensed and "medicine" consumed in private cannot be regulated by social convention. The range now covers every age group and the variety encourages experiment. There is no such thing as a harmless drug (harm is a matter of degree) yet there is no acceptable international standard for testing or comparing them, let alone legislating their use. Kids who are punished for sniffing glue out of school are fed amphetamines in class. Alcohol is totally banned, strictly rationed or actually thrust on you, depending on which country you are in; marijuana laws vary from state to state; and nobody has yet banned cigarettes, which are far more dangerous than either.

This puts an unusual degree of responsibility on the individual. More than ever it is up to you to distinguish between medical fact and political prejudice, develop a healthy skepticism of commercial pressures and mass-media hysteria, and find out what it is that you are eating, drinking and smoking – and what it will do to you.

Take care of yourself.

GENERAL

What is a drug?

A *drug* can be defined as any chemical substance taken either for medicinal purposes or socially to induce changes in perception and behavior. The difference between a drug and a food is that the former has little or no nutritional value; vitamins fall into an intermediate category, half drug and half food.

Most drugs work by affecting a particular bodily organ or tissue, or by changing general chemical processes in the body. All drugs have a large number of physical effects, some of which may only become apparent after prolonged use or above a certain dose.

This section is concerned with drugs that are commonly used (and abused) for social rather than medical reasons. It includes: alcohol, nicotine, cannabis and other hallucinogens, opiates, stimulants, and tranquilizers.

What are the main types of drugs?

Scientists usually class drugs according to their chemical composition, but the more popular classification is according to their effects. The three main types are: the *sedatives, hypnotics and narcotics*; the *stimulants*; and the *hallucinogens*. This classification is by no means complete. Nicotine, for instance, doesn't fall into any of these categories.

Sedatives, hypnotics and narcotics are all drugs which act by depressing particular or general functions in the body. Sedatives soothe anxiety and promote drowsiness. Hypnotics send you to sleep. Narcotics induce *narcosis,* a general dulling of consciousness which may vary from a mild pain-killing effect to complete unconsciousness. Many of the drugs in this overall category have all three effects, depending on the dose consumed. The category includes alcohol, the opiates (opium, morphine and heroin), barbiturates (sleeping pills), and tranquilizers. In popular terminology, they are sometimes called "downers."

Stimulants or "uppers" have the opposite effect. They induce energy and alertness, suppress the appetite, and relieve mild depression. They include caffeine, cocaine, and the amphetamines.

Hallucinogens or "psychedelic" drugs induce more or less radical changes in a person's mental state and awareness of reality. The effects vary widely from drug to drug and person to person. They include cannabis (grass, hash, THC), various kinds of mushrooms, mescaline and peyote, LSD, and a number of other synthetic chemicals. The word "psychedelic" is derived from the Greek, and means literally "making the mind clear or manifest." It is used to refer to the "mind-expanding" effects of many hallucinogens.

Why do people take drugs?

The use and abuse of drugs – for medical, social and religious purposes – is not a twentieth-century invention; it is as old as recorded history. Drugs appear to fill a human need and, if used in moderation, they by and large fill it safely.

Many drugs simply give pleasure. They induce feelings of relaxation and euphoria, or enhance one's sensual awareness of people and things. They may also be taken out of social conformity. If everyone around you smokes, or drinks, or eats magic mushrooms, you tend to follow suit. They are also a means of escape, from pain or worry or fear. The pleasures of alcohol, for instance, are largely due to its acting as a social lubricant by breaking down one's inhibitions.

Drugs can also be used out of curiosity, as a means of exploring the human potential for different states of awareness. Children all over the world seem to have a need to do this, whether by whirling around until dizzy, or sniffing glue until stoned. Drugs like the hallucinogens can be used as a means of extending one's knowledge of the world and of oneself. Priests, prophets, poets and artists have traditionally used drugs because of the insights they gain from them. Similar results can be achieved by meditation or prolonged fasting. Used in this way, drugs are a means of pushing oneself to one's physical or psychological limits.

Finally, a drug may be used because a person is addicted to it. The clearest example of this is cigarette smoking. Many smokers admit that they gain no pleasure from their habit; they simply are unable to give it up.

What is addiction? How is it caused?

Addiction is a physical condition in which a person is unable to function normally without regular doses of the drug to which he or she is addicted. Denied the drug, the person suffers unpleasant effects known as "withdrawal symptoms."

Doctors often distinguish between the above condition, which they call "true" addiction, and so-called psychological dependence. They say that some drugs have such pleasant or stress-relieving effects that the user rapidly becomes "dependent" even though physical addiction doesn't occur. To what extent "psychological dependence" is a useful category is debatable; in the context of drugs, it is often just a way of condemning the use of a drug which is disapproved of. People can become "psychologically dependent" on driving fast cars, or eating too much, or gambling, or other people. We all have our psychological crutches, and there is no scientific evidence that a non-addictive chemical is psychologically more damaging than any other type of crutch.

Physical addiction is quite another matter. It is a chronic disease which is very difficult to cure. It is often associated with "tolerance" to a drug, which means that the more of a drug you take the more you need next time to reach the same level of intoxication. Withdrawal symptoms can be extremely unpleasant, ranging from the nervousness and irritability of the smoker deprived of his next cigarette to the trembling, nausea, convulsions and delirium associated with withdrawal from alcohol, barbiturates and heroin.

Addiction is a slow process that results from the frequent consumption of a drug over a period of time ranging from months to years. Stories about people who get hooked on a drug after one or two hits are nonsense. Even in the case of heroin, addiction is a much slower process than is generally realized. And it is precisely because addiction is so gradual that many addicts, notably alcoholics, continue believing that they are not, in fact, addicted.

What causes withdrawl symptoms?

If you walk a dog at the same time every evening, it will gradually adapt so that it is ready to relieve itself at precisely that time. If you then fail to take it out one evening, it will become a very disturbed animal.

A similar process occurs when you feed your body with certain types of drug. Your metabolism and body chemistry adapt to and become dependent on the drug. Sudden withdrawal of the supply upsets the internal chemical balance you have developed. Withdrawal symptoms are the outward and sensible signs of this inner biochemical disaster.

How can I tell if I'm becoming addicted to a drug?

The symptoms of addiction vary from drug to drug, but there are several reliable indicators.

If you find yourself taking more and more of a drug over a period of time, you are in danger of addiction.

If you find yourself constantly craving another hit, you are in danger of addiction.

If you find yourself waking up in the morning with uncomfortable sensations which only your favored drug can relieve, you are in danger of addiction.

Recognizing that you are an addict is often a difficult and humiliating experience. It is also the first, vital step toward becoming cured.

Why are some drugs legal and others illegal?

The reasons are social and historical. Many legally available, over-the-counter drugs are potentially very dangerous. Cigarettes kill; aspirin is bad for the stomach; alcohol contributes to all manner of diseases, and is also a major factor in the crime statistics. By comparison, cannabis is harmless.

The distinction between legal and illegal drugs is not based on any considered scientific evaluation of the dangers involved, but on prejudice and myth. From a strictly rational viewpoint, cigarettes and alcohol should be classed with heroin as extremely addictive and hazardous substances.

It is even debatable whether *any* drugs should be outlawed. Prohibition may well cost more than lack of prohibition, and is, in any case, rarely effective. What's more, it is a virtual incitement to crime, from the bootleggers of the 1930s to the grass, cocaine and heroin smugglers of today.

In many modern western societies, the consumption of drugs on a massive scale occurs almost as a matter of course. After alcohol and tobacco, the most widely used and abused drugs are the barbiturates, tranquilizers and stimulants prescribed to millions of people to relieve stress, depression, insomnia, and other problems. People tend to feel that if they are given a drug by a doctor, it must not only be safe but positively good for them. Doctors themselves are well aware that this is not true. Many of these drugs are addictive; others may have unpleasant side effects; and in most cases, the effects of long-term use are unknown. More important, these drugs only provide temporary relief from a symptom; they do not resolve the problem that gave rise to the stress, depression, insomnia or whatever in the first place.

Illegal drugs are not somehow different from drugs prescribed by doctors, whatever the authorities or the media claim. The problem of illegal drug use is part of the overall problem of excessive drug consumption in modern societies.

ALCOHOL

Is alcohol a drug like other drugs?

Very much so. Frequent consumption over a number of years can lead to physical dependence, alcoholism, and a number of diseases. The fact that drinking alcohol is a socially acceptable form of self-intoxication in no way alters the reality that this is one of the most dangerous drugs available. It probably causes more crime, injury and death than all other drugs put together.

What is alcohol?

There are several types of alcohol, but the one used in drinks is ethyl alcohol: a colorless, volatile, inflammable and almost tasteless liquid produced by fermentation. Fermentation is a process of chemical change that occurs when living organisms such as yeast and bacteria start working on the sugars in organic substances like maize, barley, grapes, potatoes, rice, etc. While the taste of the drink varies according to the substance used, the alcohol in each is the same. Pure ethyl alcohol is also used medically as an antiseptic and a solvent.

A second kind of alcohol is methyl alcohol, also known as wood alcohol or "meths." It is used industrially as a fuel and a solvent. Extremely poisonous, its regular consumption leads to stupor, blindness and death.

How alcoholic are different drinks?

Alcoholic drinks fall into roughly two classes: those, like beer and wine, in which the alcohol is produced by fermentation alone; and the spirits, in which an additional process of distillation considerably increases the alcohol content.

Most beers and ciders have an alcohol content of up to 8 percent, most wines of 9–15 percent, and most spirits of 40–50 percent. Fortified wines and aperitifs fall into an intermediate category, and have an alcohol content of 20–30 percent.

What does "percent proof" mean?

"Percent proof" or "degrees proof" does *not* indicate the proportion of alcohol in a drink. It is a measure of the drink's specific gravity or relative density. In the US the figure for degrees proof is double the percentage of alcohol – which is why one sometimes gets bottles which are over 100° proof. Proofing regulations vary in different countries, so there is no general rule for calculating alcohol content.

What happens to alcohol in the body?

Alcohol is rapidly absorbed into the bloodstream through the linings (mucous membranes) of the mouth, stomach and intestines. Because it irritates these membranes, blood is attracted to the inflamed areas and the absorption process is accelerated. Food in the stomach reduces the irritation and thus the rate of absorption, which is why you get drunk less easily during or immediately after a meal.

Alcohol in the bloodstream acts as a mild general anesthetic, depressing bodily functions and especially the brain. Unlike some drugs which have a double action, first stimulating and then depressing, alcohol is depressive from the very first drink. The apparently stimulating initial effects result from the deadening of inhibitions and of anxiety.

Alcohol is eliminated from the body at a constant rate: about one pint of beer (two and a half bottles) or one ounce of whiskey per hour. Ten percent of it is eliminated through breathing, sweating and excreting, but the vast majority is broken down into water and carbon dioxide by the liver. Because of the slow rate of elimination, the proportion of alcohol in the blood increases rapidly during a heavy drinking session and is dissipated only very gradually. It takes your body about twelve hours to get rid of the alcohol in half a bottle of whiskey.

What are the behavioral effects of alcohol? Why do I stumble and slur my words?

Alcohol in the blood directly affects the functioning of your brain and slows down the transmission of impulses through your nervous system (which is why reflexes and reaction speed are slowed). The higher levels of the brain are dulled, releasing you from tension and worry and generating an initial sense of well-being and euphoria. As the alcohol level increases and your inhibitions break down, you may become increasingly emotional, loud, talkative and obstinate. The feeling of warmth that comes from drinking is the result of blood being diverted from your internal organs to the blood vessels in your skin. As your sensory and motor nerves become increasingly depressed and sluggish, your general physical functioning is affected: you begin to see double, slur your words and lose your sense of balance. Eventually, intoxication incapacitates you completely, and you fall into a drunken stupor; the level of alcohol in your blood at this stage is 0.30 percent, which compares with a lethal dose of about 0.60 percent.

When I'm drunk, why am I sometimes maudlin and other times aggressive?

Like many other drugs, alcohol tends to induce particular moods according to the psychological "set" of your mind at the time. The precise mechanism by which this occurs is not known; mood research is still in its infancy. But it is well known that drunks become exaggeratedly loving or violent, happy or depressed without apparent cause. Once the inhibitions that govern normal behavior are dissolved, a person's pent-up needs and frustrations tend to take over.

When I get drunk, I sometimes can't remember the next morning what happened. Why?

The occurrence of memory blackouts after a heavy bout of

drinking is commonly regarded as one of the symptoms of early alcoholism. The process that causes amnesia is unknown, but shocks to the nervous system such as concussion and heavy drinking appear to act on the brain, perhaps chemically, so that short-term memories do not get transferred to the long-term memory store. As a result, the night before remains a blank.

What causes hangovers? Can I prevent or cure them?

Hangovers are messages from your body that you have been feeding it more poison than it can cope with. The membranes of your stomach are inflamed, your body cells are dehydrated, your liver is partially incapacitated, and your nervous system is suffering from "shock." The result is headache, sensitivity to noise and light, thirst, upset stomach and nausea. While you can help to relieve these symptoms, only time can fully cure them.

Breakfast, if you can face it, will bring relief to your stomach, as will fizzy drinks. Coffee or tea will help to stimulate your depressed nervous system. Liquids will combat dehydration. Pain-relieving drugs may soothe your throbbing head, but unless you've eaten they are likely to upset your stomach even more. Some people recommend another drink – "the hair of the dog." Bloody Marys are reputed to be especially efficacious, combining nutritious tomato juice and smooth vodka. But drinking to relieve the effects of drink is like committing a second murder to cover up the first one: beware of chain reactions.

Avoiding hangovers is difficult. The best method is not to drink too much. The second best method is to eat well before or while you drink. Another method is to alternate alcoholic and soft drinks. Various types of pills (especially barbiturates), smoking, and mixing your alcoholic poisons all tend to increase the agony.

Why do some people have "weak" heads and others "hard" ones?

The answer to this question would be a major discovery. The CIA, who spent years trying to develop a pill to keep their agents from getting drunk (so that they could put the vodka-swilling opposition under the table), would like to hear from you.

The fact is that the same quantity of alcohol not only affects different people to a different extent, but also affects the same person differently on different occasions. Partly this has to do with whether you've eaten, but it is probably also dependent on the general level of your metabolism as your biorhythms move from peak to trough. It may even be affected by a lunar cycle. However, the way you react to alcohol doesn't change the amount you've drunk. Whether you are lively or comatose, you still have to cope with the same amount of liquor.

Why and how does drink affect sexual performance?

Many men use alcohol, both on themselves and on women, as if it were an aphrodisiac. It is not an aphrodisiac. What it does do is suppress your inhibitions (and maybe hers), thereby greasing the wheels of social and sexual intercourse. But alcohol does not improve sexual performance. All too often it makes sex either unsatisfactory (lack of self-control) or impossible ("brewer's droop").

Inability to get an erection after excessive consumption of beer or other alcohol is an extremely common problem, while alcoholics tend to suffer from chronic impotence.

Recent studies have shown that heavy drinking considerably reduces the production and concentration in the blood of the male sex hormone testosterone. After a month of regular heavy drinking the testosterone level is down by 50 percent.

194

This may be why chronic alcoholics tend to lose body hair, put on weight around the breasts and buttocks, and acquire other so-called "feminine" characteristics.

I believe that drinking in moderation improves my health. Is this true?

It all depends on how you define "moderation."

There is no evidence that the occasional drink does you any harm. A mealtime glass or two may improve appetite and digestion by reducing anxiety and stimulating the flow of gastric juices. The reduction of tension and worry that results from moderate drinking may make a general contribution to health as well as happiness. And the sedative effects of a bedtime nightcap may well be less physically harmful than the regular consumption of many sleeping pills. A recent study has also shown that grape juice and wine contain a chemical which reduces the activity of some gut bacteria and viruses, including the polio virus. This may help reduce your chances of infection. The study showed that white wine was more effective than red, but non-alcoholic grape juice was the most effective of all.

The traditional theory that alcohol has medicinal value if administered after shock or injury is, however, a dangerous myth. Since alcohol is not a stimulant, it serves only to depress blood pressure and other functions which are already low. Nor, according to the *Penguin Medical Encyclopedia* (1976), does alcohol help to "reduce the risk of angina by widening the coronary arteries"; improvement as a result of alcohol in such cases "is probably due to relief of worry, lower blood pressure, and diminished perception of pain."

Why does alcohol contribute to disease? What diseases can it cause?

The occasional drink may be good for you, but regular drinking to an immoderate extent is a way of poisoning yourself. The most common effects are an increase in weight, problems of the stomach and liver, and alcoholism.

Alcohol supplies the body with ready energy without providing real nutrition. It also takes precedence over food fuel, and the result is that fat and carbohydrate are stored instead of being burned. Increasing weight contributes to general ill health. More specifically, the deposition of fat instead of muscle in the heart can cause arterial problems and contribute to heart disease.

The irritation of the stomach lining by alcohol, and the pressure it puts on the functioning of the liver, can lead to gastritis and gastro-enteritis, in which the stomach and intestines become permanently inflamed; and to cirrhosis of the liver, a condition which can result in internal bleeding and the failure of the liver to function at all. The liver bears the brunt of habitual drinking, but other organs, including the kidneys, are also affected.

Alcoholism is the disease of addiction to alcohol and, if unbroken, leads to an early death. As well as having the above conditions, the chronic alcoholic is liable to suffer from vitamin deficiency, usually due to malnutrition; alcoholic myopathy, a general decay of the muscles; degeneration of the brain, involving memory loss, emotional disturbance and convulsions; and delirium tremens (the "DTs"), a state of extreme agitation often accompanied by convulsions and vivid hallucinations. Death may also result from simple consumption of an overdose; a 0.60 percent level of alcohol in the blood is lethal, causing heart and respiratory failure.

Am I in danger of becoming an alcoholic if I only drink socially? How can I tell if I'm becoming an alcoholic?

The majority of social drinkers never become alcoholics. But then the majority of alcoholics were once social drinkers who believed they would never get hooked on the stuff. Addiction is a slow and insidious process. It creeps up on you unawares, and even when you are hooked it's easy to make excuses for your habit. Recognizing that you're an addict is an extremely painful experience; it's also a necessary step to becoming cured.

If you drink in moderation and for pleasure, you're unlikely to get addicted. If you drink to relieve anxiety or stress, you may become so dependent on this alcoholic relief that you cannot function socially without it. You are then in danger of becoming physically addicted.

Early alcoholism is characterized by the urgency with which you knock back the first shot or two ("I *needed* that"); loss of memory after a heavy drinking bout; surreptitious drinking and associated feelings of guilt.

As the vicious circle tightens, the victim finds it increasingly difficult to stop drinking once he's started. He's liable to go off on alcoholic binges lasting several hours or even days. He becomes more and more obsessed and secretive, avoiding family and friends. He knows he's got a problem, but won't face up to it or ask for the help he needs. A pattern of neglect and indifference to other activities sets in. Money, work, sex, food all tend to go by the board. Abstinence from alcohol causes increasingly severe withdrawal symptoms. The man urgently requires treatment.

My work means I have to drink a lot. How can I prevent it affecting my performance?

Unless you're a professional winetaster, you don't *have* to drink at all, and you certainly don't have to drink a lot. The drinking that is conventional in many jobs is not compulsory; you won't get fired for having Coca-cola instead. Even if it did come to that, you're better off unemployed than an alcoholic.

Given all that, there are several ways of reducing the effects of drink: 1) drink slowly and drink less, 2) eat before or while you drink, 3) alternate between soft and alcoholic drinks, 4) don't mix your drinks, and don't mix drink with other drugs.

Do particular types of people become alcoholics?

Your sex, upbringing, personality, work and lifestyle all help to determine your chances of becoming an alcoholic. Men are more at risk than women, but women are catching up fast. Ten years ago the ratio of male to female alcoholics was about five to one; now about a third of all alcoholics are women. People who are emotionally or socially unstable are at risk: they tend to be the stress-relieving drinkers. Journalists, actors, executives, bartenders, salesmen and members of other "boozy" professions are at risk. The children of alcoholics are at risk. People who socialize in circles where heavy drinking is conventional are at risk.

If you don't fall into any of these categories, it doesn't mean you're not at risk. All it takes is excessive regular consumption, self-deception and irresolution.

It's a fact that doctors are more liable to become alcoholics than the members of any other profession. In Scotland, a third of all middle- and upper-class admissions to hospital for alcoholism are doctors. In the US 3 percent of all the doctors in one state were had up on alcohol-related disciplinary charges within a single decade. There's a moral there somewhere.

What can I do if I think I'm becoming an alcoholic?

You can stop drinking.

If you can't stop drinking, if you drink compulsively and suffer when you go without, then you need help. Consult your doctor.

Recognizing that you need help, and desire for help, is the first step toward becoming cured. The second step is detoxification: the process of eliminating your body's dependence on the drug. The third step is learning that you can cope satisfactorily without the drug.

Alcoholics, like other addicts, frequently go back to the bottle after supposedly being cured. This is usually because only the addiction has been treated, not the psychological problems that gave rise to addiction in the first place. Drug addiction is nearly always a psychological as well as a physical illness, and the mind needs treatment as much as the body. Plain detoxification is liable to bring only temporary relief.

One of the most important elements in kicking any drug habit is to place yourself in a situation where you will not be tempted and where you will receive constant support and encouragement. If you think you are becoming an alcoholic change your patterns of behavior and lifestyle; avoid socializing with people who drink or socialize with them at times when they don't drink; stop keeping drink in the house (or the office). Or go to Alcoholics Anonymous, whose program of mutual support through meetings and therapy sessions has proved extremely effective.

SMOKING

What are the contents of tobacco smoke? Which ingredients are addictive or dangerous?

There are three main ingredients of tobacco smoke: tar, nicotine and carbon monoxide. Each contributes to disease.

Tar is a thick brown substance formed from the solid particles in cigarette smoke. It coats the air passages down which it is inhaled, which both irritates them and prevents them from clearing themselves. It also accumulates in the lungs. It affects your breathing and can lead to bronchitis.

Nicotine is a colorless and poisonous chemical that occurs in tobacco leaves. It is believed to be the addictive ingredient of tobacco. It directly affects the nervous system. A 70 milligram injection of nicotine is a fatal dose; this compares with the 0.5–2.0 milligram nicotine content of most cigarettes.

Carbon monoxide is a poisonous gas whose effect on smokers is to displace oxygen in the blood. It can reduce the efficiency of the blood by about 10 percent, and in effect makes the regular smoker slightly anemic. The level of carbon monoxide in cigarette smoke is four hundred times the maximum allowed in factories.

As well as these major ingredients, tobacco smoke contains a large number of other chemical compounds, many of which are thought to cause or contribute to cancer.

What is "tar content?"

"Tar content" refers to the level of tar in a cigarette. It is measured in milligrams (mg) and ranges, in US cigarettes, from 2mg to 31mg. The higher a cigarette's tar content, the more damaging it is.

What do people get out of smoking?

The effects that a regular smoker experiences are minimal. There is a slight feeling of relaxation, but this is merely the result of satisfying the craving for a cigarette. Nicotine is not a relaxant drug as such. Many smokers smoke not because they enjoy it but because they can't stop. One study found that 75 percent of the smokers questioned wanted to stop, had tried at least once, but had failed.

Smoking is often used to control nervousness: it keeps one's hands occupied, and one's mouth. People smoke more when tense or anxious, but this seems to be simply a symptom of their nervousness rather than a means of relieving it. Since smoking slows one's reflexes and reactions, it is not an advantage in dangerous situations.

The first time people smoke they usually experience nausea and dizziness. Regular smokers experience a slight dizziness only after a period of abstinence. This effect is probably due to the nicotine.

Is smoker's cough dangerous?

Every time you smoke a cigarette, you add a coat of tar to your bronchial passages and lungs. The result is that the little hairs, or *cilia*, which normally clear the inhaled dirt and bacteria out of your lungs are trapped in tar and cannot perform. Pools of mucus and filth collect in your lungs as phlegm, and it is your attempts to get rid of this that causes smoker's cough. Both these gobs of phlegm and the irritation of constant coughing may cause bronchitis, which can rapidly develop into a chronic and fatal condition.

What diseases does smoking contribute to or cause?

The main types of illness caused or aggravated by smoking are respiratory disease, cancer and heart disease. The more cigarettes you smoke, the more likely you are to be affected.

The cause of smoker's cough and its contribution to bronchitis has been described above. A related illness is emphysema, in which deterioration of the lungs leads to increasingly labored breathing, to the point of causing heart failure.

Until the causes of cancer are pinpointed, no one can say just why smoking contributes to cancer. Some people have used this to argue that smoking may not cause cancer at all, and that other factors are involved. The evidence, however, is overwhelming. Smokers are seventy times more likely to contract lung cancer than non-smokers. They are also more likely to get cancer of the mouth, pharynx, larynx, esophagus, stomach and bladder.

Smoking affects the cardiovascular system generally. The lower level of oxygen and higher level of carbon monoxide in the bloodstream, the action of nicotine in constricting blood vessels and raising blood pressure, and the increase in the level of fatty acids and cholesterol in the blood, all predispose the smoker to coronary heart disease, thrombosis and harden-ing of the arteries or arteriosclerosis.

In addition to these major risk areas, smoking adds to your chances of getting ulcers, impairs your smell and taste, and reduces your appetite. Studies have shown that the children of smoker parents are much more likely to get tonsillitis, inflamed adenoids and respiratory problems than the children of non-smokers.

Will smoking shorten my life?

Every cigarette you smoke takes an average of five and a half minutes off your life, according to a recent British study. This may not seem like a lot, but at that rate someone who smokes twenty cigarettes a day loses just under two hours each day, and in a year he loses twenty-eight days, or almost a whole month. Twice as many smokers die before the age of sixty-five as non-smokers, and smokers in general have the same fatality rate as people ten years older than themselves.

Smoking kills.

Are cigars or a pipe safer than cigarettes? Is it safe to smoke five or ten cigarettes a day?

Cigar and pipe tobacco are "cured" (dried) in a different way to cigarette tobacco. Also cigar and pipe smokers usually don't inhale. These factors reduce the risks of disease, but they do *not* remove them. Because they don't inhale, cigar and pipe smokers are less likely to get bronchitis or lung cancer. On the other hand, they are more likely to get cancer of the mouth, pharynx and larynx, possibly because they absorb the nicotine through the internal linings of the mouth.

The less cigarettes you smoke, the better off you will be. But there is no safe level, and there are not many tobacco addicts who do stick to only five or ten cigarettes a day for long periods. The tendency is for one's consumption to increase imperceptibly until one finds it's impossible to manage on less than twenty a day, or thirty or forty. Far better not to smoke at all.

I know old men who've smoked forty a day all their lives and are as fit as fiddles.

This is a rare, fortunate and endangered species. Its members probably lead otherwise healthy outdoor lives in clean-air environments. They are almost certainly not as fit as fiddles.

No one knows for sure why one person will contract a disease when another, equally at risk, escapes unharmed. What is known is that smoking forty a day, or less, increases your chances of disease and early death many times over. It's not a gamble where the odds are encouraging.

Are filter tips safer than unfiltered cigarettes?

Yes, but not much. Filters are supposed to eliminate the poisonous compounds in smoke. What they in fact do is to retard them, so that they tend to accumulate in the last third of the cigarette – which is why smoking the last third, right down to the filter, poisons you more than the first two thirds. If you have to smoke, stub the damn thing out half way.

How can I give it up?

This is the desperate cry of many a smoker. The man who comes up with a sure-fire answer will be an overnight millionaire. Until he arrives, the answer is that different methods tend to suit different people. Here are a few.

Go to your doctor. Ask for help. He may suggest group sessions, hypnotherapy, aversion therapy, or other forms of treatment.

Stop dead. This is the most effective way if you are sufficiently determined and self-confident. Cutting down in the belief that you can stop completely later is usually hopeless. If you do stop dead, it helps to stay in a non-smoking environment. Keep away from smoker friends, or situations (parties, etc.) where you are accustomed to relying on the nicotine fix. Find people who will motivate and encourage you. Get a friend to give up with you so that you can mutually support each other. When you are desperate for a cigarette, do something to distract yourself: repeat a chant or rhyme, do breathing exercises, chew gum, make faces in the mirror, or read something like the last few pages which will remind you of the benefits of persevering.

Some ex-smokers say they just got up one day, looked in the mirror at their ravaged condition and never wanted a cigarette again. The majority, however, describe an arduous fight lasting weeks or months in which a constantly renewed act of self-assertion and willpower was required. Withdrawal symptoms are common: a terrible craving for a cigarette (just one, *please*), bouts of irritability, anxiety and depression.

But it's worth it. After only a few days without a cigarette you feel much better. Your cough disappears, you breathe more easily, you feel lively and cleaner in the mornings.

If you've tried to give up and failed, don't despair. Try again. Try different methods. Go to your doctor. Retire for a month to the depths of the country where the nearest cigarette is thirty miles away – the money you'll save by giving up will probably be worth any loss of income involved.

HALLUCINOGENS

What are the hallucinogens? Are they addictive?

Hallucinogens are so called because, in sufficient dosage, they cause hallucinations. Also known as psychedelic or mind-expanding drugs, their primary effect is to enhance perception and induce an altered state of consciousness. They range in intensity from cannabis to LSD.

There is no evidence that any of the hallucinogenic drugs leads to either tolerance or addiction.

I've heard about grass, hash, pot, and so on. . . . Are they all the same thing? What are the differences between them?

Cannabis or "pot" is the generic name for all the drugs derived from the plant *cannabis sativa*, also known as "hemp." The active ingredient in the plant is a chemical called THC (delta-l-tetrahydrocannabinol), which tends to be concentrated in a sticky resin secreted by the plant's flowering leaves. A long-standing myth is that only female cannabis plants produce THC, but recent studies have shown it is present in equal concentrations in plants of both genders.

Marijuana, or "grass," consists of chopped up flowers, leaves and stalks of the plant. Its potency depends partly on the source of the plant – Columbian grass and "Acapulco Gold" are reputed to be especially powerful – and partly on the proportion of flowering leaf-tops in the mixture. The word "marijuana" was first used in Mexico to refer to cheap tobacco, and only became associated with cannabis in the late nineteenth century.

Hashish or hash is made by scraping the resin from the leaves of cannabis plants and pressing the collected gooey material into solid blocks. The exact preparation varies from country to country, as does the appearance and texture of the hash. It may be light brown (Moroccan and Lebanese) or black (Nepalese and Afghan). It will also be more or less crumbly. Hash is usually mixed with tobacco to make "joints" or smoked straight in a pipe. It can also be mixed with food to make hash cookies, hash cakes, and so on.

Because it is solid resin hash is supposedly stronger than grass, but potency, in fact, varies considerably according to source and whether or not the hash has been cut with any other substance. Regular cannabis users sometimes argue that hash produces a "heavier," more drowsy kind of experience than grass, but effects vary enormously between individuals.

Although cannabis is most common in the form of grass or hash, it can also be obtained in a liquid form (hash oil) or as pills of synthetic THC.

Is pot addictive?

No. Even extremely heavy use over many years does not produce withdrawal symptoms, and the only study to find direct evidence of tolerance was one in which pigeons were given massive doses of pure THC. Pigeons aren't people.

Is it dangerous?

Nearly all the evidence suggests that cannabis is one of the safest drugs in common use. According to a standard pharmacological reference work, Goodman and Gilman's *Pharmacological Basis of Therapeutics,* "There are no lasting ill effects from the acute use of marijuana and no fatalities have ever been recorded." All the government commissions that have reported on cannabis use in the past few years have reached the same conclusion. A number of studies have suggested that cannabis can cause brain damage, but such studies involved massive dosages and were carried out on laboratory rats and cats. They are heavily outweighed by other reports showing no ill effects.

What about psychological problems as a result of cannabis use?

Abuse of any drug is sometimes a *symptom* of emotional or mental imbalance. This is not at all the same thing as a drug *causing* psychological problems. According to the British Wooton Report, published in 1968, there are no "reliable observations" in the western world of mental deterioration due to cannabis.

What cannabis can do, by sharpening the sensitivity of the user, is to exaggerate states of mind, whether of depression or elation. A paranoid person may feel more paranoid. A person on the edge of a breakdown may just be pushed over the edge. But similar effects can be caused by all manner of events and experiences, chemical or otherwise.

Another supposed danger is that cannabis use produces an "amotivational syndrome" which causes young people to "drop out" and become indifferent to conventional goals and mores. This thesis was popular when the "hippy" movement was at its height, but now that large numbers of otherwise perfectly conventional middle-class people have taken to smoking hash or marijuana it is becoming clear that any such "syndrome" is a result of complex social factors and not drug use.

What are the usual effects?

While there are thousands of individual descriptions of what it feels like to be stoned, there are very few factual studies. The result is more nonsense than sense. People's reactions to cannabis vary enormously according to dosage, personality and the situation in which they get stoned.

Two physiological changes are commonly noted: increased pulse and heart rate, and dilation of the blood vessels of the eyes (which makes the eyes very slightly redder). Subjective effects are legion: most common are a dry mouth, hunger (the "marijuana munchies") and a sharpening of the senses. Visual and auditory perception, taste, touch and smell are all intensified and/or altered. If you're extremely stoned you may experience mild hallucinations.

Cannabis can make you feel elated and giggly or relaxed and drowsy. Some people claim to think more clearly when stoned, others daydream. Some people become talkative and extroverted, others the opposite. Some feel sexier, others not. Because the effects are so variable, it is impossible to give a precise description of the experience without distortion, let alone to predict how another person will react.

One widely noted effect is "inverse tolerance" – the regular user needs less of the drug instead of more to get equally stoned. At the same time, experienced users learn to adjust to the effects and can often cope perfectly well with ordinary tasks. This was confirmed in a study by psychologist Andrew Weil, who showed that in a variety of tests, the ability of regular users to maintain attention and to perform both mental and physical tasks was not only not impaired but was sometimes actually improved. Another study compared the abilities of subjects stoned on marijuana and alcohol. Using a driving simulator, the alcohol group made many more driving errors than when sober; the marijuana group, on the other hand, performed equally well stoned and sober.

Depending on potency and the amount taken, the effects of cannabis can last from half an hour to three or four hours.

The first time I tried it, it had no effect on me. Is this usual?

This is a very common reaction. The implication is that getting stoned on cannabis is an acquired technique. It takes time to experience the full effects. Also, the effects one experiences, at least initially, may be as much due to suggestion (picked up from friends or from reading about it) as to the drug itself. This may account for the diversity of reactions. It is interesting to note that cannabis was first used medically as a mild anesthetic.

Does cannabis use lead to the consumption of "hard" drugs like heroin?

Does beer drinking lead to whiskey addiction, or eating to gluttony? No. The fact that many alcoholics started with beer and many heroin addicts with hash or grass does not mean that there is a causal connection between the two. The reasons why one person becomes an addict, of alcohol or heroin, while another doesn't, are complex and psychological.

It's sometimes suggested that because cannabis is illegal, the user must buy the drug from dealers who will also try to sell him other drugs. But this is nonsense. Most cannabis dealers do not trade in heroin and most cannabis users have no interest in heroin.

What is the legal position of cannabis?

The cultivation, possession, sale and use of all forms of cannabis are illegal in all western countries, with penalties ranging from a small fine to imprisonment. Precisely why governments spend so much time, money and manpower (police, court officials, lawyers, prison guards, etc.) in a futile attempt to suppress a harmless social habit will no doubt intrigue historians for years to come.

In the past two years or so there have been growing signs, especially in the US of a relaxation of the anti-cannabis laws. Several US states have now "decriminalized" possession of small amounts of marijuana and treat it as a minor civil offense similar to a traffic fine. And Holland is reported to be considering an approach to the United Nations to get the international drug treaty amended so that marijuana can be legalized.

What is LSD?

LSD stands for d-lysergic acid diethylamide. It was first synthesized in 1938 by Hoffman and Stoll at the Sandoz pharmaceutical company in Switzerland, but its effects weren't discovered until Hoffman took some accidentally in 1943 and went on the first ever "acid trip." It was used primarily for medical and research purposes (including by the CIA) until the mid-1960s, when the work of Timothy Leary and the "acid tests" of Ken Kesey and his Merry Pranksters introduced it to popular use.

LSD is one of the tryptamine group of hallucinogenic drugs, which includes psilocybin and DMT. It is a derivative of ergot, a type of fungus which grows on rye. Outbreaks of ergot poisoning due to infected crops may have been partly responsible for the dancing hysteria in medieval Europe.

LSD is one of the most potent drugs known. The usual illegal dose is 100–300 micrograms, or *millionths* of a gram. Quantities as small as 1/700 millionth of a person's body weight are sufficient to induce hallucinogenic effects, and three ounces of LSD would be sufficient to affect a million people.

On the black market, LSD is usually available in pill form. It can also be obtained as a powder or liquid; dissolved onto sugar cubes or blotting paper; or as minute squares of transparent gelatine ("window-pane" acid).

What are the effects of LSD?

Just how LSD affects body and brain chemistry is unknown. Most of the drug concentrates in the liver, kidneys and adrenal glands, with only about 1 percent in the brain – but it is this 1 percent that seems to produce the strongest effects. There is an enormous literature on LSD experiences. Everyone who has taken acid has his or her own tale to tell, and each person's reactions tend to be unique. What follows is therefore a summary of the most common effects.

LSD begins to act about half an hour after ingestion, and the trip lasts from six to twelve hours, depending on dosage. The effects tend to come in waves of increased intensity, with relatively less intense periods in between.

The first and most notable effect is enhanced visual perception. On acid, you see *more*: more color, more texture, more shapes and patterns. It is as if you have never before fully appreciated the object or person you are looking at. Moreover, you don't just see things "in a new light," you feel that you are seeing them as they really are, without the habits of thought and emotion which normally cloud your perception. Similar changes occur with your other senses: you hear more, taste more, feel and smell more. In the more intense stages of the trip, this increased perception develops into proper hallucinations, especially visual ones, as if you are dreaming while wide awake.

The LSD user typically remains fully aware that he is hallucinating. He doesn't imagine, as the hallucinating alcoholic often does, that what he is seeing is really there. Indeed, experienced acid users can often control their reactions and switch back to "normal" vision when they want to. Hallucinations tend to occur periodically throughout the trip, diminishing in frequency and intensity as the effects of the drug wear off.

While the perceptual effects are common to nearly all users, the emotions and ideas they evoke in a person are extremely variable. On some occasions, you may have ecstatic, mystical-type experiences; other times, you may go through the terrors of a "bad trip." A relatively common element in the latter is the feeling that you have lost control of yourself and have no ability to affect what happens to you and how you react. The more frightened you become, the more out of control you feel. This can lead to a feeling of loss of identity, as if you are dissociated from yourself.

The unpleasantness of this experience may simply be due to your fighting against what you are feeling. In a good trip, similar feelings are enjoyed and built on. It is largely a question of attitude. The feeling of loss of identity that is so terrifying in a bad trip is converted, in a good trip, into a sense of union with Nature or God, of "oneness" with the universe.

Your reactions to other people may be equally extreme, ranging from feelings of isolation and paranoia to a sense of being incredibly close to and at one with friends, loved ones, or even strangers. However, acid trips are by no means always so extreme.

Acid can also be used as a means of exploration. You can control to a certain extent what you pay attention to. LSD becomes a kind of psychic microscope with which you can investigate your body or mind, or other people's, or the world about you. Because habitual patterns of perception, thought and behavior are eliminated, such exploration often leads to powerful insights which may be retained long after the trip is ended.

Finally, one's sense of time during a trip is completely distorted. It's a bit like living in slow motion. Because of the intensity of experience what, in fact, takes only a few seconds may seem like minutes or hours.

An acid trip leaves one mentally exhausted, and ready for a long deep sleep.

What about sex on acid?

Timothy Leary claimed that LSD was the most potent aphrodisiac ever discovered, while anti-LSD propagandists have told lurid tales of innocent young women drugged into wild orgies. Most authors, however, have reached much less spectacular conclusions. Acid does not seem to be a physical aphrodisiac in the sense of impelling one to have sex; what it does do is radically alter one's experience of sexual intercourse, enhancing tactile and other perceptions and the feeling of communion with one's partner.

What causes a bad trip? Can I prevent it? What can I do about it if I'm having one?

There's no certain answer to what causes a bad trip, and no guaranteed means of preventing one. What you experience on acid is probably determined by the total circumstances in which you take LSD, including your background and character, your mental, physical and emotional state, and the events of the trip itself. Several situations should be avoided: tripping when you are depressed, anxious or under stress; tripping in unfriendly or unfamiliar places; tripping alone or with people you cannot trust to look after you. None of these circumstances guarantees a bad trip, but it may predispose you to having one.

Once you are into a bad trip, the only certain cure is time – but anything that serves to distract you, to make you feel that the trip will improve, or will end quickly, is recommended. Powerful tranquilizers act as antidotes to LSD and help bring to an end. Some people believe that orange juice also helps. But the best thing of all is to have one or more friends who, preferably, are not tripping themselves and who can "talk you down." Patient and friendly reassurance that your situation is improving, that the trip will end soon, that you are indeed loved and not isolated (or whatever your particular terror may be) will soothe the unpleasantness. A bad trip is a matter of getting trapped in a vicious circle of fear.

Is LSD psychologically dangerous?

Acid trips are nearly always extremely powerful experiences, emotionally and mentally. Like other such experiences – grief, love, religious conversions, close brushes with death – they can radically alter one's idea and behavior for a longer or shorter period. Anything this powerful is *potentially* dangerous, and *is to be treated with care.*

There are good trips and bad trips, and bad trips can induce feelings of paranoia, schizophrenia, and mental instability. But there is no firm body of evidence to indicate that a bad trip will permanently affect an otherwise healthy individual. The "experts" disagree. One problem is that there have been very few studies of normal LSD use (as opposed to CIA and US Army studies of its use under interrogation or battle conditions). Another problem is that a number of the studies have been biased. One study that revealed "psychotic" reactions to LSD turned out on closer analysis to have involved a number of subjects who had previously been under psychiatric care. In such cases, an LSD trip can obviously trigger off "psychotic" reactions, as can a great many other things.

Cases have been reported in the media of people on acid being blinded because they stared too long at the sun; being run down because they imagined they could halt traffic by holding up a hand; and, an old favorite, plunging to their deaths while under the delusion that they could fly. There is very little hard evidence to back these stories. The blindness case was traced by the Canadian Government Commission of 1970 to a hoax fabricated by an American state official. And there is only one well-documented case of someone trying to fly while on acid.

Other stories implicate LSD and other hallucinogens in the commission of violent or bizarre crimes. The Manson murders were said to have been committed on acid. Other murderers have claimed to be on acid when they did the foul deed, and that they were therefore not responsible for their actions. Such stories are hearsay. There is no evidence linking LSD use with crime. Indeed, the weight of the scientific evidence favors the view that LSD increases feelings of warmth and comradeship and reduces feelings of hostility. Someone who is already hostile and aggressive may be triggered into action by LSD, but he is far more likely to be triggered off by alcohol – as the statistics linking drunkenness and crime amply show.

Because there is no firm data on how many people use LSD, and how often, no one knows what proportion of trips are bad ones. But since doctors and psychologists, in fact, tend to see only the bad cases, there is probably a natural tendency to exaggerate their frequency.

One final point: it *is* dangerous to give someone LSD without telling them, since they are only too likely to think, when the effects begin, that they are going crazy.

Does LSD cause any physical damage?

Some scientific research has suggested that LSD use can damage your chromosomes and cause genetic mutations. The case, however, is far from proven. In the first place, several of these studies involved fruit flies or rats who were given massive LSD injections. In the second place, chromosomal damage in humans can be caused by many other factors, including radioactivity, some virus infections, and even aspirin and caffeine. Finally, other studies have revealed no link between LSD use and such damage.

What is notable is that there is no suggestion of any other physical damage caused by LSD. However, no one has the first idea what long-term effects might be caused by regular use over a long period. All drugs should be taken with caution.

What about flashbacks?

Flashbacks are the spontaneous return of a state of consciousness or an hallucination associated with a drug. Though most commonly noted with LSD, they also occur with other drugs, including cannabis. They may occur days, months or even years after the drug was taken. They are also probably quite rare. The number of LSD flashbacks reported is not large, though this may be because most flashbacks are not sufficiently unpleasant to induce the person to go to a doctor.

What causes flashbacks is unknown, but since they can occur so long after an acid trip they are almost certainly not physical in origin – LSD is eliminated from your body in a matter of hours. The fact that they are usually very specific, involving the recurrence of a particular experience or hallucination, also suggests that the mechanism is psychological. Some scientists have suggested that they may be triggered off by an idea or perception associated with the original experience, rather like epileptics whose fits appear to be triggered by a particular smell or taste.

Flashbacks need not be unpleasant; it depends what is flashed back to, and the situation in which the flashback occurs. Their unexpectedness, however, is likely to be disconcerting, and can be dangerous.

What are peyote and mescaline?

Peyote is a small, grayish-brown, spineless cactus that grows in the arid parts of northern Mexico, and is used as a psychedelic substance by a number of Mexican and American Indians. The usual method is to cut the cactus top into slices which are dried and chewed as peyote or mescal "buttons." The taste is said to be extremely unpleasant, causing nausea and vomiting, as well as hallucinogenic effects.

Peyote contains a number of psychedelic ingredients, of which mescaline is one. Nowadays, mescaline is usually manufactured in a laboratory. Its name is derived from the Mescalero Apaches. Its modern use was popularized by Aldous Huxley, whose description of its effects in *The Doors of Perception* is still the most complete.

The usual mescaline dose is about 500 milligrams, and is taken in pill form. The effects start about an hour after ingestion and last from four to twelve hours. The trip can be terminated, or alleviated, by taking a powerful tranquilizer.

The mescaline trip is similar to the LSD trip, though experienced users of both usually say that mescaline is less harsh or "artificial" in its effects, and more mellow and "organic." To what extent this difference is due to auto-suggestion is impossible to judge. Certainly, there are fewer reports of bad trips on mescaline, but then the drug is much less widely used than LSD. Nor is it certain how much of the mescaline sold on the black market is the real thing; where analysis has been done, "mescaline" has often turned out to be LSD or other hallucinogens.

What other hallucinogens are there?

Psilocybin is a derivative from the mushroom *Psilocybe Mexicana*, or "magic mushroom." The active element is chemically similar to but less potent than LSD. The drug can be obtained either in synthetic or mushroom form. The trip lasts four to twelve hours and is similar to LSD and mescaline trips.

Fly agaric (*Amanita muscaria*) is another psychedelic mushroom, with a red top and white spots. It was once used as fly poison. The active ingredients include two hallucinogenic agents, atropine and bufotenine. It induces sweating, nausea and a much reduced heart rate as well as psychedelic effects.

DMT is a semi-synthetic drug chemically similar to psilocybin and produces a mild LSD-type experience that lasts only half an hour; as a result it was dubbed "the businessman's lunchtime high," though it's doubtful whether any executives were involved.

STP is a synthetic and naturally occurring chemical which is related to both mescaline and amphetamine. The trip is said to resemble the imagined effects of imbibing liquid rocket fuel, and one theory has it that STP is an acronym for Scientifically Treated Petroleum. In fact, petroleum doesn't come into it. The chances of a bad STP trip are said to be considerable.

OPIATES, STIMULANTS BARBITURATES AND TRANQUILIZERS

What are the opiates?

The opiates are a group of drugs derived from opium, which is the dried juice from seeds of the Indian poppy. They include morphine, codeine and heroin. They act by depressing the central nervous system, and especially affect the senses, reducing pain and promoting sleep. As such, they have been and still are widely used as painkillers and sedatives. In larger doses, however, they act on the pleasure centers of the brain and produce dreamy feelings of serenity and euphoria. All the opiates create tolerance and physical addiction after prolonged regular use.

Opium has been used for centuries in Asia and the Middle East. The poppy juice is prepared in either liquid or powder form, and is traditionally smoked in a pipe.

Morphine is the main active ingredient in opium, and is ten times stronger. It is mainly used as a painkiller.

Codeine or methyl morphine is a mild opiate used with aspirin to treat headaches. Because of its low potency, massive doses would be needed to induce pleasurable effects or addiction.

Heroin is described below.

Is heroin as dangerous as it is claimed to be?

Heroin, also known as smack, horse or H, is usually billed as the most dangerous of all drugs, and the heroin addict as the most sinister, twisted and dangerous of addicts. There is so much myth and fear surrounding heroin abuse that it is difficult to find any rational discussion of the subject.

Heroin is three times more potent than morphine. It was first produced in 1898 and was intended, ironically, as a powerful but non-addictive painkiller. On the black market, it is obtained in the form of a white powder which can be "snorted" up the nostrils or injected. The latter method is preferred by most addicts because it produces an immediate and powerful rush of euphoria, followed by intense feelings of pleasure and contentment. Most black market heroin is cut with other substances, such as baking powder or talc, and is therefore far from pure. Variations between the potency of heroin bought on the street is one reason why addicts frequently overdose themselves.

There is a widespread belief that heroin is instantaneously addictive: take it once and you're hooked. This is nonsense. Like other drugs of addiction, physical dependence results only from regular and prolonged use. Just how quickly a person becomes addicted will depend on his constitution, the regularity with which he takes it, the dose he takes and the reason why he takes it. Some people may become addicted in a matter of weeks, but in other cases it takes months or years. In *Drug Dependence* (Faber, 1970), J.H. Willis mentions that hospital patients may be given heroin once every few days for over a year without becoming addicted. It may be that the sense of craving for and dependence on the drug common among junkies accelerates the addiction process.

Every form of addiction is a disease which is both physically damaging and difficult to cure. But there is no evidence that heroin addiction is any worse, physically, than addiction to alcohol or barbiturates. Many of the ills from which junkies suffer are the result of the life they lead rather than the heroin itself. Use of unsterilized hypodermics is a common cause of infection.

It is often said that heroin addiction causes crime. What, in fact, causes crime is the junkie's need to acquire the large sums necessary to support his habit. The penniless addict suffering from acute withdrawal symptoms will indeed resort to almost anything to get his next fix, but as many American law enforcement officers recognize, it is the law rather than the drug which causes this situation. In Britain, where registered addicts can get their supply cheaply and legally on prescription, the junkie crime problem hardly arises. It's also the case that the vast profits in the smuggling and sale of heroin have traditionally attracted the criminal underworld, from Chinese Triads to American Mafia.

Breaking a heroin habit is difficult and painful. Hospital treatment often involves giving the addict an alternative drug – methadone or tranquilizers – to help him through the withdrawal period. But this can lead to dependence on the alternative. As with alcoholism, the desire to be cured and a completely drug-free environment both during and after withdrawal are vital.

What is speed?

Speed refers to drugs of the amphetamine type and is so called because they induce activity, wakefulness and talkativeness, together with a general sense of self-confidence and well-being. They are also known as "uppers."

There are many types of amphetamine, but the most common in illegal use are various pills (Benzedrine, Dexedrine and methedrine) and a powder (amphetamine sulphate). Sulphate can either be snorted or injected the latter method providing an immediate "rush" beloved of the "speed freak." Amphetamines are prescribed medically to suppress appetite (i.e. in some diet pills), to keep people awake, and to alleviate mild depression.

Speed works by stimulating the central nervous system. The physical effects include increased heart rate, blood sugar and muscle tension. Amphetamine drugs are similar to the hormone adrenalin which is produced in the body at times of stress, fear and excitement.

Regular and constant use of speed eventually leads to both tolerance and physical addiction. The speed freak may go for several days without food or sleep, with consequent physical deterioration. He is liable to garrulousness, feelings of paranoia and bouts of depression after large doses. Overdoses cause death; as the well-known phrase puts it, "speed kills."

What is cocaine?

Cocaine or "coke" is a white crystalline powder obtained from the cocoa plant in Columbia and Peru. Like the amphetamines, it induces wakefulness, alertness of mind, mild euphoria and loss of appetite. It is also a local anesthetic, and has been used as such in medicine and dentistry. Back at the turn of the century, Coca-cola used to contain a small amount of cocaine – hence its name. What we drink now is certainly not "the real thing."

Cocaine can be injected or snorted. Constant snorting, though the most common method, can eventually damage the linings of the nostrils and the bridge that separates them.

Cocaine is classified in most western countries as a "hard" drug of addiction. The *Penguin Medical Encyclopedia* (1976) describes it as "notorious" and addictive, habitual use leading to "grave deterioration of personality and sometimes frank insanity." This assertion is contradicted by most authorities, who agree with J.H. Willis in *Drug Dependence* that "there is no physical dependence." Evidence for mental instability as a result of cocaine use is rare and mainly anecdotal. In general, the drug's effects are mild and pleasant. The stories of cocaine addiction may well be derived from Sherlock Holmes' notorious liking for a "seven percent solution" of the drug, of which Watson violently disapproved. Holmes was, however, a fictional character.

As with cannabis and LSD, the supposed dangers of cocaine are almost certainly exaggerated. A recent report about its consumption by Indians in the Andes, who chew the leaves of the cocoa plant, suggests that it is a valuable addition to their low-protein diet because it keeps up blood glucose levels and slows down the break-up of blood sugar. For the Indians at least, it is both food and drug.

What about barbiturates and tranquilizers?

After alcohol and cigarettes, barbiturates and tranquilizers are the most commonly used drugs in western societies. The barbiturates – seconal, nembutal, tuinal, etc. – are commonly prescribed as sleeping pills. However, there is now growing recognition in the medical profession that they are among the most dangerous drugs available, leading to severe physical addiction and occasional death by overdose, especially if mixed with alcohol.

Tranquilizers, by comparison, are relatively safe. They are known as the "benzodiazepine" group of drugs, and include Valium, Librium, Mogadon, and other famous brand names. They are not addictive.

Both barbiturates and tranquilizers work by depressing the central nervous system, but they often induce a brief initial feeling of euphoria before drowsiness takes over. Like alcohol, however, they tend to diminish a person's inhibitions against aggression and can, paradoxically, lead to violent behavior. A Canadian study found that the prescription of tranquilizers to prisoners increased rather than decreased violent behavior; and there is also evidence that tranquilizer consumption is common among women who batter their babies. Such problems are only beginning to be recognized. Most doctors, and all drug companies, argue that the benefits of tranquilizers outweigh the dangers.

Aging

Old age is a cultural definition not a biological one. We don't suddenly become old at some arbitrary age like sixty or seventy. Yet our society treats old age as a frontier beyond which you become an irrelevant nuisance. We have covered some of the physical changes which aging brings about, but they are nothing compared to the psychological problems caused by lack of self-respect and the feeling of uselessness once we have crossed the threshold of retirement. Boredom and frustration can shorten a life more effectively than arthritis.

If you worry about it beforehand you are likely to put it out of your mind, which only compounds the problem when you finally have to face up to it. But if you plan ahead, refuse to accept the labels tied on you, involve yourself with other age groups and see old age as a continuation of the present rather than a break with the past, it becomes something to look forward to. Far from being a depressing period, it can be the most fruitful ten, twenty or even thirty years of your life.

"Age only matters when you are aging," said Picasso. "Now that I have arrived at a great age, I might just as well be twenty." And Picasso was not unique in that respect. Tolstoy, Churchill, Ghandi, de Gaulle, Michael-angelo, Yeats, Verdi, Freud, Frank Lloyd Wright, Sophocles, Grandma Moses, Jung and Mao Tse Tung – and many others – achieved their finest when they were over sixty, and so can you.

GENERAL

What causes aging?

The short answer is that no one knows for sure. Aging is one of the major mysteries of modern biology. Doctors and scientists, however, have plenty of ideas. Their theories fall into two basic categories. One school argues that aging is a built-in process: we grow old because we are programmed to grow old by our genes. It isn't in the interest of the species for individuals to live too long; if they have lived long enough to reproduce they have fulfilled their basic genetic task.

The second school of thought holds that aging is just the result of "wear and tear." In theory we could live forever, but in practice the stresses and strains of life, both physical and psychological, cause our bodies to run down.

The currently favored villain of the "wear and tear" theorists is the process of cell mutation. Nearly all body cells reproduce by dividing into two at regular intervals, so as to replace cells that have died. In the course of a lifetime, however, many cells may become damaged or subject to mutation. Diseases, toxic chemicals, radioactivity, exposure to X-rays and to the sun's ultraviolet radiation, are all known to cause cell damage and mutation. The gradual accumulation of mutant and damaged cells, this theory suggests, weakens and eventually disrupts the efficient operation of body tissues and organs. In the case of cancer, mutant cells actively attack and take over parts of the body.

Another factor which many people agree contributes to aging is stress. Intense grief, fear, pain or anxiety can all make a person "old before his time." But the biological mechanisms underlying such changes are unknown.

Improvements in diet, hygiene and medical science have all contributed to extending western man's average lifespan. This has increased both the proportion of old people in the population, and the length of time most of us spend in "old age." It is probable that the emphasis in medical research will shift in the future from extending human life to extending human youthfulness.

When does aging begin? When do I become "old?"

As a process of gradual physical degeneration, aging begins in your middle or late *twenties*, and continues until death. It is therefore wrong to pick out a particular age – such as sixty or sixty-five – as marking the onset of "old age." Different people age at different rates. Even more important, they age in different ways. Some men (and women) retain a relatively youthful appearance even as they grow old in spirit; others may have wrinkles and white hair, and still be as sprightly as men many years younger.

"Old age" is not just a condition of the body; it is also an attitude of mind. The inner man counts as much, probably more, than the outer appearance. You don't suddenly "become old" at a particular age or when your hair turns gray, or when you retire from work, or when you start thinking and feeling old. In this sense, there are old men of thirty and young men of ninety.

Why do some people age faster than others? What is the normal rate?

The rate at which you age may result from inherited problems, from the kind of life you lead, or from both these factors.

Certain habits and lifestyles are well-known causes of premature aging: an insufficient or badly balanced diet; excessive use of cigarettes, alcohol or other addictive drugs; lack of physical hygiene and care; overwork; lack of physical and mental exercise; emotional and mental stress.

Both disease and sudden shock can make a person appear to age almost overnight. But here as elsewhere, appearances are often deceptive. The outward appearance of age doesn't necessarily reflect the inner biological degree of aging.

As for the "normal" rate of aging, there is *no* normal rate. There is a spectrum of rates, and even this spectrum varies according to how you define aging – is it white hair, or loss of muscle strength, or decreasing brain weight, or declining heart-lung capacity? Trying to decide whether you're aging faster or slower than average is a futile exercise. The answer is almost certainly that in some ways you are aging faster, in others slower, and the less you worry about it the longer you'll stay young.

What happens to my body as I get older?

As you grow older, your body loses weight, strength and flexibility. Your muscles become smaller and weaker, your joints less easily articulated, and your bones more brittle. Speed, force and ease of movement are all reduced. Most of your internal organs – heart, lungs, liver, kidneys – become smaller and less efficient. A seventy-five-year-old man's heart has only about 70 percent of the output of a thirty-year-old's; his kidneys are only 60 percent as efficient; and his maximum oxygen uptake during exertion is only 40 percent.

Your arteries grow harder and narrower with age, causing a gradual increase in blood pressure. At the same time, the flow of blood to the brain is reduced and this, together with the loss of nerve cells, probably accounts for much of the slowing of brain function associated with old age.

Your senses slowly become duller. Vision and hearing become less acute. And by the age of seventy-five, you have only one third of the taste buds you had at thirty. At the same time, the slowing down of your brain functioning impairs your ability to interpret and respond to sensory stimuli.

These gradual changes, and others too, result in two overall effects. First, your body is unable to do as much as when you were younger. Your maximum work rate at the age of seventy-five is only about 70 percent of when you were thirty; even more significant, your maximum work rate in a short burst (such as an emergency) is only 40 percent of when you were thirty.

The second major effect is that your body has less reserve capacity, and you are consequently less able to resist and recover from disease, cope with a crisis, or regain equilibrium after stress. In other words, as you grow older you live much closer to your physical limits than when you were young. This loss of flexibility is one of the key characteristics of aging.

Is it true that I get smaller and lighter as I get older?

Yes. Your height declines by at least 2–3 inches as you age. There are two causes. First, your spine becomes slightly shorter because the vertebral discs deteriorate. Secondly, the weakening of your body muscles means that you can no longer hold yourself as erect as before. It is this loss of posture that is responsible for most of the loss of height.

Your weight also declines gradually from about the age of sixty. By the time you are seventy-five, you will probably weigh about 88 percent of what you did when young. This loss of weight is primarily due to loss of tissue: muscles, organs, bones are all smaller and lighter. However, if you experience any sudden and unexplained weight loss, you should consult a doctor since it may be a symptom of disease.

The loss of weight with age is both small and very gradual.

Why does the skin wrinkle with age?

As you grow older, the dead cells that make up the outer layer of your skin, or *epidermis*, are replaced more slowly by new cells from the layer below. The result is that your outer skin tends to become scaly and cracked. At the same time the inner layer of skin, or *dermis*, shrinks and loses its elasticity. The fatty content of the dermis is reduced, causing a general loss of bulk. And the sweat and oil glands, which have kept your skin soft and smooth, secrete less – so that your skin becomes dry.

Frequent exposure to the sun adds to the dryness of your skin. In spite of their overall fitness, ski instructors usually have the wrinkled appearance associated with old age when they are still in their forties and fifties. Delaying wrinkles is a matter of skin care throughout your life.

Once they have appeared, wrinkles can only be removed by cosmetic surgery, an expensive and sometimes painful procedure recommended only for the extremely vain.

SEX AND FITNESS

How does growing old affect the sexual urge?

Sexual activity and potency decline with age, but this may well be due more to social and psychological limitations than to physical ones. A fit and healthy man should, in theory, be able to have intercourse at any age.

As you grow older, your production of the male sex hormone, testosterone, decreases steadily. This decline starts when you're about twenty and continues all your life. In about 95 percent of men, however, the amount of testosterone produced, even in very old age, is sufficient for sexual intercourse.

Another factor affecting sexual activity as you grow older is your general physical decline. As you lose youthful strength and energy, the physical processes of sex – semen production, erection, ejaculation – tend to slow down and to require added stimulation.

In most cases, therefore, the physical process of aging is only a minor factor in the decline of sexual activity with age. The most common causes, in fact, are lack of opportunity and lack of potency.

Impotence doesn't necessarily involve any loss of desire for sex. Indeed, it is frustrating and humiliating precisely to the extent that one wishes for sex but cannot, for one reason or another, succeed in it.

The percentage of impotent men rises rapidly after the age of fifty. The reasons for this are extremely varied – tiredness, drink, depression, difficulties with one's partner – and have already been dealt with. Age can also provide men with an excuse for ending sexual relations which have become routine or which make them anxious.

Lack of a partner can also be a major difficulty, as can the "dirty" image that sexual activity between older people, or between an older and a younger person, has acquired.

Is there a male menopause?

This is a matter of some controversy. Most doctors and psychologists define "menopause" in a narrow, physical sense as the changes in hormone production and ending of menstruation that occur in women in their middle or late forties. Though 1 or 2 percent of men do undergo a similar experience, with a sudden reduction in their production of the male sex hormone and consequent loss of potency, the vast majority of men have no physical equivalent of the female menopause.

Many people, however, define "menopause" much more

loosely to describe the "change of life" that comes when you realize you are growing old, losing your sexual attractiveness, and that your youthful dreams may remain forever unfulfilled. The associated feelings of depression are then described as "menopausal." Some men, in fact, develop physical menopausal symptoms: not only impotence, but also hot flushes like those experienced by many women. Most doctors suggest that the latter are psychosomatic, produced in imitation of the female experience.

The problem with describing bouts of middle-aged anxiety and depression as a male menopause is that it implies they are a natural, and even inevitable, occurrence. If you get depressed or lose your potency at this time of life, you can blame it on your age and your hormones and make no effort to understand or deal with it further. Middle-aged impotence, however, is a relatively common complaint that may be caused by a large number of different factors, and which may arise aged thirty-five, forty-five or fifty-five. It is *not* "menopausal."

Nor are bouts of depression menopausal, whether accompanied by impotence or not. Life is full of bouts of depression, from teenage identity crises to feelings of futility or despair when you retire from work. Dignifying bouts of middle-aged depression with pseudo-medical titles like "male menopause" is often an excuse for not facing up to what is really troubling you.

Is it wrong for older men to be attracted to younger women or girls? If I feel such an attraction, will people think I'm a "dirty old man?"

Whether you're sixteen or sixty, to be physically attracted to an attractive women is a natural part of being a heterosexual male. There's nothing in your genes that programs you to stop being attracted to women when you reach a certain age, or to be attracted only to women of roughly your own age. On the contrary, both social conditioning and genetic programming conspire to make younger women seem more attractive than older ones.

Straightforward attraction is not the only reason. Many older men get enormous satisfaction from knowing that they are still sufficiently "virile" to interest a young woman or girl. Equally, there are young women who are especially attracted to older men. There is nothing wrong about such attractions, or about sexual relations resulting from them, as long as both partners are consenting.

It is nonetheless true that a sexual relationship between a young woman or girl and a much older man gives rise to gossip, and often to jealousy and malice. It is difficult, but best, to ignore this. The phrase "dirty old man" is a term of abuse on a par with "filthy nigger" and should be treated as a symptom of the prejudice and ignorance of the person who uses it.

It is unfortunately true that the different age groups in modern industrial societies are becoming increasingly segregated. The young have little opportunity nowadays to see and learn what older people are really like. The resulting ignorance fosters superstition and myth. Age prejudice is as invidious as race prejudice.

Can sexual intercourse or masturbation endanger my heart?

If you are just about to have a heart attack, it's possible that an active bout of sex will trigger it off. But so might any other form of exertion.

If you are seriously worried that your sexual activity could affect your health, consult your doctor. There's no point in giving up one of the major pleasures in life on the basis of an unconfirmed anxiety.

What about sports or other types of exercise?

Regular and moderate exercise, even at an advanced age, strengthens the heart and contributes to overall good health. Indeed, lack of exercise among middle-aged and older people allows muscles to grow weak, joints stiff, and the circulation sluggish – all of which contribute to cardio-vascular or rheumatic problems in old age.

The most important things about exercise in old age are that it should be regular (daily) and moderate. Violent, sudden or prolonged exercise can be dangerous. So start and finish gradually. Do not push yourself "until it hurts," and stop immediately if you experience any pains, or shortness of breath or pounding of the heart.

If you have been inactive for a long time, and decide to take exercise at an advanced age, consult your doctor first.

How can I stay fit in old age? Are there special types of exercise?

Some old people are as fit and vigorous as many a younger man. This is usually the result not of strenuous training programs, but simply of daily physical activity or exercise. As you grow older, the more violent forms of sport will place too great a strain on your body – especially competitive sports in which you may force yourself to greater exertion than is good for you. But activities like swimming, cycling, walking and gardening; and sports such as golf and even tennis, can be enjoyed by those accustomed to them up to an advanced age.

Exercise can also be taken indoors. Indeed, perhaps the most important element in exercise as you grow older is that you should put all your muscles and joints through a full range of movement every day. Stretch all your muscles, especially when you wake up in the morning or after a rest. All the joints should also be fully exercised – neck, shoulders, elbows, hands, hips, knees and feet. Such a daily regimen will maintain your muscle tone, joint flexibility and posture. There are various sets of exercises, from traditional calisthenics to yoga, which provide a full complement of routines. Consult a physical education or other relevant teacher, especially if you plan to start after a period of inactivity.

There are also special exercises which help to alleviate or prevent particular medical conditions, including certain heart problems and some forms of arthritis. These will be prescribed for you by a doctor or physiotherapist.

PROBLEMS OF AGE

Is it normal to sleep less as you grow older?

Older people not only tend to sleep for less time, they also sleep more fitfully, often waking several times a night. This disturbed pattern of sleep can lead to feelings of tiredness and listlessness during the day. Many old people go to bed earlier, get up later, and take an afternoon rest as well, in spite of sleeping for less time. A vicious circle is likely to arise: the more you rest during the day, the less you are likely to sleep at night and the more tired you'll feel the next day.

Mundane factors also contribute to sleeplessness. Old mattresses may be hard and uncomfortable, and you may feel their discomforts more as you get older. Too many or too few covers may leave you uncomfortably hot or cold. And tea or coffee before bedtime may keep you awake.

One solution is to take a sleeping pill, but this also has its problems. As mentioned, some sleeping pills (the barbiturates) are addictive, and may also make you confused or affect your memory when you're awake. Sleeping pills also tend to suppress the dreaming process, giving you an inferior quality of sleep and possibly causing emotional or mental problems.

A far healthier solution than a sleeping pill is to take enough exercise in the course of the day to make you gently tired.

What causes painful joints? Is there a cure?

Painful joints, especially in old age, are almost certainly due to one of the diseases generally known as rheumatism or arthritis. Most of these diseases are ill-defined and poorly understood. Treatment is often restricted to painkillers, which relieve the symptoms but do not solve the problem. There are three main types that affect older people: osteoarthritis, rheumatoid arthritis, and gout.

Osteoarthritis seems to be an almost inevitable consequence of aging. It affects 80 to 90 percent of people over sixty, and men more than women. It involves degeneration of the cartilage which acts as a kind of washer between the bones in a joint. The cartilage loses its elasticity, and may begin to break up. The joint becomes swollen and painful. The bones harden and may develop rough deposits and spurs. The problem tends to affect the joints which have been most subject to wear and tear in your life: usually the knees, hips or hands. There is no known cure. Painkillers can relieve the agony, and gentle, regular exercise can prevent the joints becoming stiff. In extreme conditions, surgery may help. The joint can even be replaced altogether by a metal ball and socket.

Rheumatoid arthritis involves the inflammation of the connective tissue around a joint, especially the knuckles and wrists. Typically, a tender knot or nodule of tissue forms just under the skin. The problem often begins in late middle age, becoming more severe as you grow older. In most cases an attack subsides after a while, though it may recur over and over again. Sometimes there is a persistent, aching inflammation in which the affected joint becomes increasingly stiff and, in very severe cases, dislocated or crippled. The cause of the disease is unknown. Special exercises and painkilling drugs are the main forms of treatment.

Gout is a disease involving sudden and sharp pains in a joint (proverbially the big toe). It is caused by the accumulation in the joint of crystals of uric acid. These crystals are in turn attacked by phagocytes, which are part of your body's defense system, and it is the release of toxic substances by the phagocytes which appears to cause the actual symptoms of gout. Contrary to myth, gout is not entirely due to excessive drinking, though alcohol can trigger off and aggravate an attack. A change of diet (and abstention from alcohol) helps to control but will not cure gout. A number of drugs are available, however, which serve either to relieve an attack or to prevent the accumulation of uric acid crystals between attacks.

What is hypothermia?

Hypothermia is a state of extreme body cold, and occurs when the body temperature falls below the normal 95°–99°F. It is most common amongst older people who cannot afford adequate food, clothing and heating. As his temperature falls, the hypothermia victim grows more and more lethargic. He may be unaware of his plight, although his body is cold to the touch, even in normally warm places like the armpits. Below 90°F coma usually occurs, and death follows.

Rewarming the hypothermia victim should be done gently and slowly. Sudden or direct application of heat can be dangerous; so can a "medicinal" shot of alcohol. The room should be warmed gradually, and the patient wrapped in a blanket and given warm (not hot) coffee, tea or soup. A doctor should be called.

How does aging affect eyesight?

The most important effect is *presbyopia*, the hardening of the lens of the eye with age. This loss of elasticity begins at about the age of ten. By the time you're sixty, it has significantly reduced your ability to focus on things close up, and you will tend to hold a book or newspaper further away. Short-sighted people may suddenly find that they can read without their glasses, but in most people the opposite is the case: glasses become necessary for reading or other close-up work.

Older people should have their eyes checked once a year, both to keep track of their presbyopia and to ensure early detection of such problems as cataracts and glaucoma.

What is a cataract?

Cataract is a disease in which the lens of the eye becomes increasingly opaque, causing dimness and eventually loss of vision. It usually occurs in people over the age of fifty to sixty and is a gradual process which affects one eye more than the other. Early symptoms include seeing double (when sober), fixed (rather than floating) spots in front of the eyes, and a general deterioration of eyesight.

Operations to remove a cataract are now routine and effective. They are performed under local or general anesthetic, and involve a one- or two-week stay in hospital. Afterward, eyeglasses with one strong lens have to be worn, and may take a little getting used to, but sight is almost fully restored.

What is glaucoma?

Glaucoma is a condition usually occurring in old people in which the pressure of the fluid in the eye (the *aqueous humor*) increases slowly or suddenly and disturbs the eyesight. If untreated, it leads to blindness.

Acute or sudden glaucoma involves sudden intense pain in one eye accompanied by extremely blurred vision, nausea and vomiting. It requires emergency admission to hospital, but is very rare. The much more common chronic type, on the other hand, produces no apparent symptoms and may pass unnoticed until severe damage to the eye has already occurred. This is one reason why it is vital to have your eyes checked annually as you get older.

The precise cause of glaucoma is uncertain, but if caught in time it can be treated with drugs or by surgery.

How does aging affect the hearing?

The onset of deafness with age is a slow and insidious process which is partly due to reduced sensitivity of the ears, and partly to other communication difficulties that old age brings, such as slowness of comprehension and inability to listen attentively. Deafness is also one of the least understood of the disabilities of age and often causes a degree of impatience and irritation in others which is an added affliction to the sufferer.

The most common effect of age on the hearing is loss of the ability to distinguish high-pitched sounds. By the age of sixty, hearing of these is reduced by 75 percent. The result is often infuriating since spoken consonants fall in this high-pitched range and are thus very difficult to distinguish. When you ask the person to repeat what he said, he assumes you are deaf and raises his voice. This does nothing to improve your perception of consonants. And if you then exclaim, "There's no need to shout, I'm not deaf," the circle of mutual incomprehension is complete.

The solution to this common problem is to explain your difficulty right at the start. You can hear most things perfectly well, but find it difficult to distinguish consonants. Would the person you are talking to please speak directly to you (so that you can see his lips), talk slowly, and enunciate his or her words distinctly.

The inability to distinguish high-pitched sounds is one

example of *perceptive deafness*, in which sounds are difficult to interpret because they are distorted. Perceptive deafness is usually a problem of the inner ear and the brain, and is not solved by raising the volume. *Conductive deafness*, on the other hand, is what people normally think of as deafness: a reduction in the loudness of the sound perceived. It is usually due to infection or blockage of the outer or middle ears, which conduct the sound waves to the inner ear. Accumulation of plugs of ear wax are one cause of conductive deafness. Other forms can be treated surgically or with various medicines. And hearing aids can be used to amplify the sound.

What about hearing aids?

Hearing aids consist of a microphone, an amplifier and an ear-piece, and they are usually specially molded to fit snugly into your ear canal.

Straightforward amplification of the sound reaching your ear can often overcome the problem that causes conductive deafness. In most cases of perceptive deafness, however, the hearing aid simply makes you more aware of unintelligible noise, though in some cases a hearing aid can help by picking out and amplifying particular types of sound.

As well as the common type of hearing aid described above, and known as an *inset receiver*, there are also *flat receivers* and *bone conductors* which are prescribed when an insert is ruled out by some ear condition.

What is Parkinson's disease? Can it be cured?

Parkinson's disease or *parkinsonism* is a condition in which muscles grow rigid and give rise to involuntary twitching and trembling movements. The onset of the disease is gradual. A frequent early symptom is difficulty in controlling one's handwriting. As the muscular rigidity spreads, it makes movement difficult and sluggish. Walking becomes a shuffle, speech may become slurred, and stiffness of one's facial muscles may give one a rigid, masklike appearance. Though these symptoms lead many people to imagine that the victim of Parkinson's disease has become moronic, intellectual faculties, in fact, remain unimpaired.

The disease results from degeneration of a particular part of the brain, the basal ganglia, which controls voluntary movement. The cause of the degeneration is uncertain, but the drug L-Dopa has been found to relieve the symptoms of the disease in 75 percent of cases.

Parkinson's disease affects men more than women. It is named after James Parkinson (1755–1824), a London physician.

What causes incontinence? Can anything be done about it?

Incontinence is the inability to control one's bladder or bowels, and is one of the most humiliating of the physical problems associated with age. In most cases, however, both urinary and fecal incontinence are of a *temporary* nature, caused by disease or emotional stress. Once the cause is cleared up, continence returns. It is only in a minority of cases that incontinence is chronic and beyond remedy.

Urinary incontinence is frequently associated with infections in and around the bladder, including stones and prostate gland trouble. Constipation can also be a cause, as can certain drugs which encourage urination or which relax the muscles. Since incontinence can often be a symptom of some infection, it is important to report it to the doctor as early as possible, in spite of any embarrassment you may feel.

In many older people, urinary continence is only precariously maintained, and a sudden shock or upset such as a bereavement or anxiety, can temporarily disturb it.

Fecal incontinence is most often due to prolonged constipation. A mass of feces, too bulky and hard to be passed, accumulates in the rectum and interferes with your muscle control. This impacted mass acts like a ball valve, allowing fresh feces to escape in a continuous trickle. Treatment involves removal of the offending mass. Fecal incontinence may also be caused by diarrhea or by conditions affecting the brain, such as a stroke.

SENILITY

What is senility? What are its causes?

Senility is not a word describing any precise medical condition. It is a popular word that refers to overall changes in mental and emotional functioning in old age. These changes include deterioration of intellectual faculties like memory and comprehension; changes in temperament and personality that range from apathy and melancholia at one extreme to a "second childhood" at the other, and changes in behavior due to mental or physical restrictions.

To what extent such changes are due to the physical process of aging is extremely uncertain. Social and psychological deprivation is certainly just as important as physical deterioration. Another factor is medical mistreatment, especially the overprescription of drugs. These causes are dealt with in turn below.

What physical changes contribute to senility?

One of the most dramatic changes in your body as you grow older is the loss of nerve cells. By the age of seventy, your brain weighs only half what it did when you were thirty. This is because brain cells, unlike other body cells, do not divide and replicate; when they die, they are not replaced.

But the effect of this brain cell loss is extremely uncertain In the first place, the human brain has a great deal of spare capacity. In the second place, its effective functioning probably depends on more complex factors than simply the number of brain cells. The fact is that some people have active minds at one hundred years old when others begin to deteriorate at sixty. So it seems that something more than straightforward nerve cell loss is required to cause serious impairment to a particular mental faculty or to mental activity in general.

This additional factor is in many cases faulty blood supply to the brain. Hardening, narrowing and blocking of the arteries can lead to a gradual or, in the case of a stroke, sudden decline in the blood reaching the brain. This deprives the brain of its vital supplies of oxygen, either generally or locally, which is why a stroke can all of a sudden deprive you of speech or paralyze your limbs. When the decline in blood flow and oxygen supply is more gradual and less localized, the effects are not so dramatic: gradual loss of memory; increasing forgetfulness; disorientation in time and space; blunting of the perceptions and emotions; confusion, apathy and listlessness. These symptoms may increase in severity almost imperceptibly over a period of years.

Another physical factor that can affect mental functioning is disease in other parts of the body. Even among younger people, certain diseases may cause mental confusion or emotional distress. In older people, these effects tend to be more acute.

To put these problems into perspective, only 10 percent of people over sixty-five, according to one estimate, have any organic brain disorder.

What about social and psychological factors?

Old age frequently involves a radical change in a man's status and style of life at a time when he is physically and psychologically ill-equipped to meet the challenge.

Retirement after a lifetime of work may involve loss of income and feelings of uselessness, depression and boredom. Social isolation may result from being cut off from one's workmates, and also from reduced mobility and the death of friends or relations. Declining physical capacity may make one increasingly dependent on others. Old people are often made to feel unwanted. They are given no role to fulfill, no sense of purpose. The pace of modern life may leave them frightened and bewildered.

It is little wonder that some respond with listlessness, apathy, irritability or eccentric behavior – symptoms which are taken as signs of physical degeneration and senility. But this isn't senility; it is the avoidable psychological (and medical) cost of a callous social structure.

Physical and psychological causes of "senility" interract. Illness or physical disability contribute to a person's depression, while depression may prolong or even bring on an illness or disability.

What about medical factors?

Certain forms of treatment, and especially the prescription of large numbers of drugs, may themselves be a major cause of mental confusion and other symptoms of senility. A recent survey of elderly patients admitted to a hospital in Manchester, England, showed that 10 percent were there as a direct result of drugs prescribed by doctors, and that an astonishing 62 percent had been prescribed drugs in unnecessarily large quantities. Two patients admitted for *senile dementia* – a loss of reasoning power, memory and will – made a remarkable recovery when taken off the tranquilizer Largactil. One had been prescribed the drug because his doctor thought he was disturbed when, in fact, he was desperately worried about acute constipation. The other was suffering from mild confusion because of narrowing of the arteries in the brain, but was made much worse by the drug.

Whether the Manchester survey is representative of practice in the rest of England, let alone the US is uncertain. It is nonetheless true that elderly patients are often prescribed so many pills that even a computer couldn't predict the possible side effects. Most drugs arc, in any case, tested for side effects on young and middle-aged people, not older ones. Zut older people, because of physiological changes, may react different-ly to a particular drug or combination of drugs. Older people also tend to have a lower tolerance. They may suffer from physical or psychological effects which a younger person might shrug off.

The implication is that mood-altering drugs such as tranquilizers, anti-depressants, sleeping pills and stimulants should be taken with extreme caution. Unfortunately, even doctors cannot be relied upon in this area.

BIBLIOGRAPHY

Peter Wingate, *The Penguin Medical Encyclopedia* (Penguin, 1976).

Solid, useful and comprehensive, this is a basic non-technical reference work. Entries are informative and succinct, and cover everything from athlete's foot to heart surgery. They describe both the symptoms of diseases, their causes (where known), and the orthodox forms of treatment.

The Diagram Group, *Man's Body* and *Woman's Body* (Paddington Press, 1976).

Quite simply the best, most straightforward and most useful reference books about the human body. Easy to read, excellently laid out, and with a large number of informative diagrams and illustrations.

Russell L. Rhodes, *Man at His Best* (W.H. Allen, 1975).

Subtitled "How to be more youthful, virile, healthy and handsome," this book is aimed at the junior executive type. It covers such subjects as appearance, fitness, weight control, body odor, and some aspects of sex. There are chapters on physical exercises and diets. There are also some extraordinary sketches showing you how to keep fit while sitting at your office desk (when your secretary's not looking.) Mr. Rhodes maintains that both business success and a happy social life depend on an attractive appearance.

Charles Hix, *Looking Good: A Guide for Men* (Hawthorn Books, 1977).

Packed with pretty photographs of male models, this is a kind of male *Vogue* which projects a macho, ultra-cool, playboy image. Recommended only for the truly vain. Mr. Hix has apparently spent many years writing about male grooming, and his text is so groomed as to be positively unreal.

Anthony Pietropinto and Jacqueline Simenauer, *Beyond the Male Myth* (Times Books, 1977).

The results of the first major survey on male sexuality since Kinsey, although not in the same league as the original. The style is jokey, but the 4,000 essays and interviews based on a list of forty questions provide a mass of fascinating information and quotations. If you want to know where you stand on love (25.2 percent said they could lead a full life without it), having sex during a woman's period (31.4 percent said it made no difference), delaying your orgasm (14.7 percent said they didn't bother), or monogamy (only half said they would be satisfied with it), or a welter of equally subjective subjects, then this is where you can check out the averages.

Barry McCarthy, MD., *What You (Still) Don't Know about Male Sexuality* (Thomas Crowell Company, 1977).

This is a well-written account of sexual psychology with lots of practical advice on fears, anxieties and other problems. In spite of the facetious title, there is no sensationalism, statistics or special pleading for the latest "cult" theory – just casebook examples and a sympathetic, good-humored text that makes you want to keep on reading.

Philip. R. Roen, MD., *Male Sexual Health* (William Morrow and Company Inc., 1974).

A non-technical question-and-answer book with diagrams. Mainly concerned with the prostate and addressed to the middle-aged likely to be having their first problems with it.

Gilbert Cant, *Male Trouble: A New Focus on the Prostate* (Praeger Publishers, 1976).

The latest treatment, drugs and surgery by an ex-medical editor of *Time*.

Michael DeBakey and Antonio Gotto, MD., *The Living Heart* (David McKay Company Inc., 1977).

An immensely detailed and authoritative account of modern heart surgery by two famous specialists, with fascinating stitch-by-stitch diagrams of all the main operations. But the text is heavy with technical jargon and not for beginners.

Paul Kezdi, MD., *You and Your Heart* (Atheneum/SMI, 1977).

Practical advice on how to avoid heart disease by modifying your lifestyle. A fluent text with a few judicious (and frightening) statistics and details of the latest theories and research. The best $10-worth of health insurance you could buy.

Andrew Weil, *The Natural Mind* (Jonathan Cape, 1973).

One of the most thought-provoking and readable introductions to modern illegal drug use, from cannabis to LSD. Dr. Weil is one of the world's leading authorities on marijuana, and has written an eminently careful and sensible book.

Solomon H. Snyder, MD., *Uses of Marijuana* (Oxford University Press, 1971).

An in-depth look at the medical and social uses of cannabis, its history, behavioral and physiological effects and potential dangers.

D.B. Bromley, *Psychology of Human Aging* (Viking, 1974).

The best introduction to the problems of old age.

INDEX